KT-568-926

ABC of
Interventional Cardiology

Second Edition

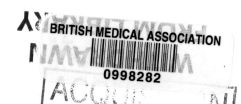

ABC series

An outstanding collection of resources - written by specialists for non-specialists

The *ABC* series contains a wealth of indispensable resources for GPs, GP registrars, junior doctors, doctors in training and all those in primary care

- **Now fully revised and updated**

- **Highly illustrated, informative and a practical source of knowledge**

- **An easy-to-use resource, covering the symptoms, investigations, treatment and management of conditions presenting in day-to-day practice and patient support**

- **Full colour photographs and illustrations aid diagnosis and patient understanding of a condition**

For more information on all books in the *ABC* series, including links to further information, references and links to the latest official guidelines, please visit:

www.abcbookseries.com

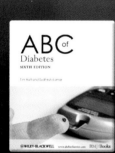

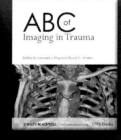

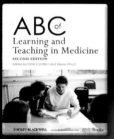

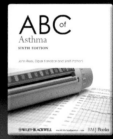

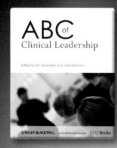

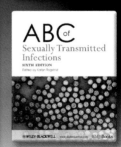

WILEY-BLACKWELL

BMJ|Books

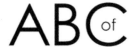

ABC of
Interventional Cardiology

Second Edition

Ever D. Grech

Consultant Cardiologist
South Yorkshire Cardiothoracic Centre, Northern General Hospital, Sheffield, UK

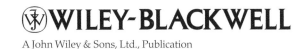

WILEY-BLACKWELL

A John Wiley & Sons, Ltd., Publication

BMJ|Books

This edition first published 2011, © 2011 by Ever D. Grech
Previous edition: 2003

BMJ Books is an imprint of BMJ Publishing Group Limited, used under licence by Blackwell Publishing which was acquired by John Wiley & Sons in February 2007. Blackwell's publishing programme has been merged with Wiley's global Scientific, Technical and Medical business to form Wiley-Blackwell.

Registered office: John Wiley & Sons Ltd, The Atrium, Southern Gate, Chichester, West Sussex, PO19 8SQ, UK

Editorial offices: 9600 Garsington Road, Oxford, OX4 2DQ, UK
                 The Atrium, Southern Gate, Chichester, West Sussex, PO19 8SQ, UK
                 111 River Street, Hoboken, NJ 07030-5774, USA

For details of our global editorial offices, for customer services and for information about how to apply for permission to reuse the copyright material in this book please see our website at www.wiley.com/wiley-blackwell

Library of Congress Cataloging-in-Publication Data

ABC of interventional cardiology / Ever D. Grech. – 2nd ed.
       p. ; cm.
    Includes bibliographical references and index.
     ISBN 978-1-4051-7067-3 (pbk. : alk. paper)
   1. Heart – Diseases – Treatment. 2. Coronary heart disease – Surgery. I. Grech, Ever D.
   [DNLM: 1. Cardiovascular Diseases – therapy. WG 120]
   RC683.8.A33 2010
   616.1′2 – dc22
                                           2010039150

ISBN: 978-1-4051-7067-3

A catalogue record for this book is available from the British Library.

Set in 9.25/12 Minion by Laserwords Private Limited, Chennai, India

Printed in Singapore by Ho Printing Singapore Pte Ltd.

1   2011

Contents

List of Contributors

Abdallah Al-Mohammad

Consultant Cardiologist, South Yorkshire Cardiothoracic Centre, Northern General Hospital, Sheffield, UK

Kevin S. Channer

Professor of Cardiovascular Medicine, Royal Hallamshire Hospital, Sheffield, UK

Ever D. Grech

Consultant Cardiologist, South Yorkshire Cardiothoracic Centre, Northern General Hospital, Sheffield, UK

Julian Gunn

Senior Lecturer and Honorary Consultant Cardiologist, University of Sheffield, Sheffield, UK

Gerald C. Kaye

Consultant Cardiac Interventional Electrophysiologist, Princess Alexandra Hospital, Woolloongabba, Brisbane, QLD, Australia

Damien Kenny

Specialist Registrar in Paediatric Cardiology, Bristol Royal Hospital for Children, Bristol, UK

Laurence O'Toole

Consultant Cardiologist, South Yorkshire Cardiothoracic Centre, Northern General Hospital, Sheffield, UK

Jonathan Sahu

Consultant Cardiologist, South Yorkshire Cardiothoracic Centre, Northern General Hospital, Sheffield, UK

Robert F. Storey

Reader and Honorary Consultant Cardiologist, University of Sheffield, Sheffield, UK

Kevin P. Walsh

Consultant Paediatric Cardiologist, Our Lady's Hospital for Sick Children, Dublin, UK

Preface

It is only 33 years since the first percutaneous transluminal coronary angioplasty (PTCA) was carried out by the pioneering Swiss radiologist Andreas Greuntzig in Zurich, heralding the dawn of interventional cardiology. In this short time, interventional cardiology has overcome many limitations and undergone major evolutionary changes – most notably the development of the intracoronary stent and more explicitly the drug-eluting stent. Across the world, many thousands of patients now safely undergo percutaneous coronary intervention everyday and the numbers continue to grow. In many countries, the numbers far exceed surgical bypass operations.

Although at first, PTCA was indicated only as treatment for chronic stable angina caused by a discrete, easily accessible lesion in a single coronary artery, this has now progressed enormously to encompass complex multi-lesion and multi-vessel disease. Moreover, percutaneous coronary intervention has now become widely used in the management of acute coronary syndromes (which principally include 'heart attacks') with definite benefits in terms of morbidity and mortality. The effectiveness and safety of these procedures has undoubtedly been enhanced by the adjunctive use of new anti-platelet and anti-thrombotic agents, and newer drugs are being evaluated. As drug-eluting stents address the Achilles' heel of angioplasty and stents – restenosis – the huge increase in percutaneous coronary procedures seen over recent years is likely to continue.

As the indications increase and more patients are treated, so inevitably do the demands on healthcare budgets. Although percutaneous intervention is expensive, this burden must be weighed against bypass surgery which is significantly more costly and multi-drug therapy which would be required over many years.

Although percutaneous coronary intervention has held centre stage in cardiology, major in-roads have also been made in non-coronary areas. Transcatheter valvular treatments – including actual new valve implantation, closure devices and ethanol septal ablation – have become effective and safe alternatives to surgery, as have paediatric interventional procedures. A greater understanding of cardiac electrophysiology and heart failure has led to important advances in the treatment of arrhythmias and resynchronisation therapy. Pacemakers, implantable cardioverter defibrillators (ICD) and cardiac resynchronisation therapy (CRT) are benefiting ever larger numbers of patients both in terms of life quality and mortality.

Where are we heading? This is perhaps the biggest question in the minds of many interventional cardiologists. New ideas and technology generated by industry, coupled with high levels of expertise, are fuelling advances in almost all areas of interventional cardiology. The next decade promises many new (and possibly unexpected) developments in this exciting and restless field of medicine.

In writing this book, I have endeavoured to present broad (and sometimes complex) aspects of interventional cardiology in a clear, concise and balanced manner. To this end, I have concentrated on an easy-to-read style of text, avoiding jargon and exhaustive detail where possible and supplemented with many images and graphics.

Ever D. Grech
Sheffield

Acknowledgements

I have many people to thank for their help in developing and producing this book. I am very grateful to my co-authors who have all willingly contributed their time and expertise. I would also like to recognise the positive efforts and invaluable assistance of the editors and publishers at Wiley-Blackwell. These include Laura Quigley, Adam Gilbert, Carla Hodge and Karen Moore. My thanks also to Dhanya Ramesh at Laserwords.

Finally, my enduring gratitude goes to my wife Lisa and our children Alexander and Frances for their unfailing encouragement, patience and love.

List of Abbreviations

CTO	Chronic total occlusion
HRT	Hormone replacement therapy
IVUS	Intravascular ultrasound
LAD	Left anterior descending (artery)
LCx	Left circumflex (artery)
Non-STEMI	Non-ST segment elevation myocardial infarction
PCI	Percutaneous coronary intervention
RCA	Right coronary artery
STEMI	ST segment elevation myocardial infarction

List of Trial Abbreviations

ACE	Abciximab and Carbostent Evaluation
ADMIRAL	Abciximab before Direct Angioplasty and Stenting in Myocardial Infarction Regarding Acute and Long-Term Follow-up
ASSENT-4	Assessment of the Safety and Efficacy of a New Treatment Strategy for Acute Myocardial Infarction
BARI	Bypass Angioplasty Revascularisation Investigation
CADILLAC	Controlled Abciximab and Device Investigation to Lower Late Angioplasty Complications
CAPITAL-AMI	Combined Angioplasty and Pharmacological Intervention Versus Thrombolytics Alone in Acute Myocardial Infarction
CAPTURE	C7E3 Antiplatelet Therapy in Unstable Refractory Angina
CARDia	Coronary Artery Revascularisation in Diabetes
CARE-HF	Cardiac Resynchronization – Heart Failure
CARESS-in-AMI	Combined Abciximab REteplase Stent Study in Acute Myocardial Infarction
CHAMPION	Cangrelor Versus Standard Therapy to Achieve Optimal Management of Platelet Inhibition
CHARISMA	Clopidogrel for High Atherothrombotic Risk and Ischemic Stabilization Management and Avoidance
CLARITY	Clopidogrel as Adjunctive Reperfusion Therapy
COMMIT	Clopidogrel and Metoprolol in Myocardial Infarction Trial
COMPANION	Comparison of Medical Therapy, Pacing, and Defibrillation in Chronic Heart Failure
COURAGE	Clinical Outcomes Utilising Revascularisation and Aggressive Drug Evaluation
CREDO	Clopidogrel for the Reduction of Events during Observation
CURE	Clopidogrel in Unstable Angina to Prevent Recurrent Events
ECSG	European Cooperative Study Group
EPIC	Evaluation of C7E3 for Prevention of Ischemic Complications
EPILOG	Evaluation in PICA to Improve Long-Term Outcome with Abciximab Glycoprotein IIb/IIIa Blockade
EPISTENT	Evaluation of Platelet IIb/IIIa Inhibitor for Stenting
ESPRIT	Enhanced Suppression of the Platelet Glycoprotein IIb/IIIa Receptor Using Integrilin Therapy
EUROPA	European Trial on Reduction of Cardiac Events with Perindopril in Stable Coronary Artery Disease
EVEREST	Endovascular Valve Edge-to-Edge Repair Study
FAME	FFR Versus Angiography for Multivessel Evaluation
FINESSE	Facilitated Intervention with Enhanced Reperfusion Speed to Stop Events
FREEDOM	Future Revascularisation Evaluation in Patients with Diabetes Mellitus: Optimal Management of Multivessel Disease
FRISC II	Fast Revascularisation during Instability in Coronary Artery Disease
GISSI	Gruppo Italiano per to Studio della Sopravvivenza nell'infarto miocardico
GUSTO	Global Utilization of Streptokinase and Tissue Plasminogen Activator for Occluded Coronary Arteries
GUSTO IV ACS	Global Use of Strategies to Open Occluded Arteries IV in Acute Coronary Syndrome
HOPE	Heart Outcomes Prevention Evaluation
HORIZONS-AMI	Harmonizing Outcomes with Revascularization and Stents in Acute Myocardial Infarction
ICTUS	Invasive Versus Conservative Treatment in Unstable Coronary Syndromes Investigators

IMPACT II	Integrilin to Minimize Platelet Aggregation and Coronary Thrombosis
ISAR-COOL	Intracoronary Stenting with Antithrombotic Regimen Cooling Off
ISAR-REACT 2	Intracoronary Stenting and Antithrombotic Regimen – Rapid Early Action for Coronary Treatment 3
ISIS-2	Second International Study of Infarct Survival
JUPITER	Justification for the Use of Statins in Prevention: an Intervention Trial Evaluating Rosuvastatin
MADIT I and II	Multicenter Automatic Defibrillator Implantation Trials. The Use of Defibrillators in Primary Prevention
MIST	Migraine Intervention with Starflex Technology
MUSTT	Multicenter Unsustained Tachycardia Trial
On-TIME 2	Ongoing Tirofiban in Myocardial Infarction Evaluation
PARAGON	Platelet IIb/IIIa Antagonism for the Reduction of Acute Coronary Syndrome Events in the Global Organization Network
PEACE	Prevention of Events with Angiotensin-Converting Enzyme Inhibition
PLATO	Platelet Inhibition and Patient Outcomes
PRISM	Platelet Receptor Inhibition in Ischemic Syndrome Management
PRISM-PLUS	Platelet Receptor Inhibition in Ischemic Syndrome Management in Patients Limited by Unstable Signs and Symptoms
PROSPECT	Predictors of Response to Cardiac Resynchronization Therapy
PURSUIT	Platelet Glycoprotein IIb/IIIa in Unstable Angina: Receptor Suppression Using Integrilin Therapy
RAPPORT	Reopro and Primary PTCA Organization and Randomized Trial
RAVEL	Randomised Study with the Sirolimus-Eluting Velocity Balloon-Expandable Stent in the Treatment of Patients with De Novo Native Coronary Artery Lesions
RESTORE	Randomized Efficacy Study of Tirofiban for Outcomes and Restenosis
RITA 3	Randomised Intervention Treatment of Angina
SCD-Heft	Sudden Cardiac Death in Patients with Heart Failure
SHOCK	Should We Emergently Revascularize Occluded Coronaries for Cardiogenic Shock
SIRIUS	Sirolimus-Coated Velocity Stent in Treatment of Patients with De Novo Coronary Artery Lesions Trial
Stent-PAMI	Stent Primary Angioplasty in Myocardial Infarction
SYNTAX	Synergy between PCI with Taxus and Cardiac Surgery
TACTICS-TIMI 18	Treat Angina with Aggrastat and Determine Cost of Therapy with an Invasive or Conservative Strategy – Thrombolysis in Myocardial Infarction
TAMI	Thrombolysis and Angioplasty in Myocardial Infarction
TIMI IIIB	Thrombolysis in Myocardial Infarction IIIB
TRANSFER-AMI	Trial of Routine Angioplasty and Stenting after Fibrinolysis to Enhance Reperfusion in Acute Myocardial Infarction
TRITON-TIMI 38	Trial to Assess Improvement in Therapeutic Outcomes by Optimizing Platelet Inhibition with Prasugrel – Thrombolysis in Myocardial Infarction
TRUCS	Treatment of Refractory Unstable Angina in Geographically Isolated Areas without Cardiac Surgery
VANQWISH	Veterans Affairs Non-Q-Wave Infarction Strategies in Hospital
VINO	Value of First Day Coronary Angiography/Angioplasty in Evolving Non-ST Segment Elevation Myocardial Infarction
WHO MONICA	World Health Organisation: Monitoring Trends and Determinants in Cardiovascular Disease

CHAPTER 1

Modifying Risk Factors to Improve Prognosis

Kevin S. Channer[1] *and Ever D. Grech*[2]

[1]Royal Hallamshire Hospital, Sheffield, UK
[2]South Yorkshire Cardiothoracic Centre, Northern General Hospital, Sheffield, UK

OVERVIEW

- Certain personal characteristics and lifestyles point to increased likelihood of coronary heart disease and are called *risk factors*

- The three principal modifiable risk factors are smoking, hypercholesterolaemia and hypertension. Other modifiable factors linked to lifestyle include a saturated-fat-rich diet, obesity and physical inactivity

- Prevention strategies (primary or secondary prevention) aim to reduce the risk of developing or retard the progression of atheroma, to stabilise plaques and to reduce the risk of their erosion or rupture. These measures can collectively reduce the risk of future cardiovascular events (mortality, myocardial infarction and strokes) by as much as 75–80%

- Percutaneous coronary intervention (PCI) or coronary artery bypass graft (CABG) revascularisation is not a cure for coronary heart disease and they are predominantly carried out to improve symptoms. They may have little or no prognostic impact in chronic stable angina. However, CABG and PCI confer significant short- and long-term mortality benefit in acute coronary syndromes and, in particular, primary PCI for acute ST segment elevation myocardial infarction

Table 1.1 Risk factors for the development of premature ischaemic heart disease and acute myocardial infarction.

Risk factor	RR*	Modifiable	Not modifiable	RR for AMI†	PAR for AMI (%)†
Smoking	5.1	√	–	2.87‡	35.7‡
Age	4.7	–	√	–	–
Abnormal lipids	3.1	√	–	3.25	49.2
Hypertension	3.1	√	–	1.91	17.9
Diabetes	2.0	√	–	2.37	9.9
Male sex	2.0	–	√	–	–
Obesity	1.8	√	–	1.12	20.1
Positive family history	1.5	–	√	–	–
Psychosocial factors	–	–	√	2.67	32.5
5× daily fresh fruits/vegetables	–	√	–	0.70	13.7
Regular alcohol	–	√	–	0.91	6.7
Regular exercise	–	√	–	0.86	12.2

Uncertain risk factors include: hypertriglyceridaemia, lipoprotien (a), microalbuminuria, uric acid, renin, fibrinogen, C-reactive protien and hyperhomocyteinaemia.
*From Steeds. RR, Relative risk.
†From INTERHEART case-control study. Yusuf S *et al. Lancet* 2004;**364**: 937–52.
‡For current and former smokers.
RR for AMI: Relative risk for acute myocardial infarction. PAR for AMI(%): Population attributable risk for acute myocardial infarction.
Notes: These 9 risk factors accounted for 90% of the population attributable risk in men and 94% in women. Psychosocial factors included depression, stress at work or at home, moderate/severe financial stress, one or more recent life events, low control score. The control population was drawn from hospital in-patients with non-cardiac conditions (58%) and community-based hospital visitors (36%). A minority were WHO MONICA controls (3%) and unknown (3%).

In affluent societies, coronary artery disease causes severe disability and more deaths than any other disease including cancer. It manifests itself as silent ischaemia, angina, unstable angina, myocardial infarction, arrhythmias, heart failure and sudden death. Although this is the result of atheromatous plaque formation and its effect, the actual cause of this process is not known. However, predictive variables – known as *risk factors* – have been identified which increase the chance of its early development. Risk factors can be classified as modifiable and non-modifiable (Table 1.1).

It is clearly not possible to prevent the increased risk associated with ageing, a positive family history or male gender. However, there are many factors which can be usefully ameliorated by interventions. Moreover, there are some aspects of lifestyle that have been shown to reduce the risk of an acute myocardial infarction.

ABC of Interventional Cardiology, 2nd edition.
© Ever D. Grech. Published 2011 Blackwell Publishing Ltd.

Risk factors are not simply additive but may be synergistically cumulative. Data from epidemiological surveys have shown for some time that combinations of risk factors generate exponential risks (Figures 1.1 and 1.2). This applies to both men and women. Risk factors are not static but increase with age – this may partly explain the independent effect of age. Blood pressure increases normally with age, so whatever definition is used for hypertension, the frequency of this condition will increase with age. Cholesterol and triglycerides increase with age as do insulin resistance and body mass index.

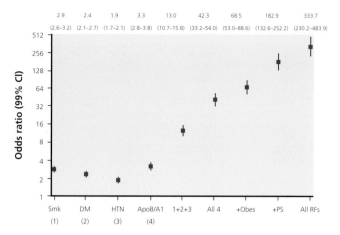

Figure 1.1 The adverse effect of single and combined risk factors on the risk of acute myocardial infarction. Smk, smoking; DM, diabetes mellitus; HTN, hypertension; ApoB/A1, lipid abnormalities; Obes, obesity; PS, psychosocial factors; RFs, risk factors. From INTERHEART case-control study. Yusuf S *et al. Lancet* 2004;**364**:937–52.

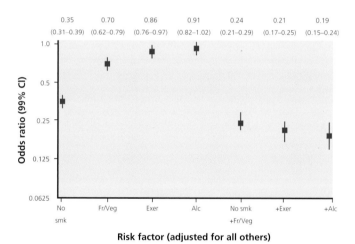

Figure 1.2 The beneficial effect of single and combined risk factors on the risk of acute myocardial infarction. No smk, no smoking; Fr/Veg, daily 5 fresh fruits/vegetables; Exer, regular exercise; Alc, regular alcohol. From INTERHEART case-control study. Yusuf S *et al. Lancet* 2004;**364**:937–52.

Impact of risk factors

Smoking

Smoking confers a fivefold relative risk for acute myocardial infarction and cardiovascular death. By comparison, stopping smoking has an almost immediate effect on reducing the cardiovascular risk by about 50%. Ex-smokers still have a higher risk than lifelong non-smokers. In one study, the survival rate of patients who stopped smoking after an acute myocardial infarction at 8 years of follow-up was about 75% compared with 60% for patients who continued to smoke. Similarly reinfarction is about twice as common in smokers than in those who stop smoking after a first infarction. At 8 years of follow-up, reinfarction was about 38% in smokers compared with 22% in quitters. Overall smoking increases mortality by about 2.5 times and reduces absolute survival by, on average, 10 years.

Hyperlipidaemia

High blood cholesterol is associated with an increased cardiovascular risk. However, as a single risk factor it is relatively weak – it becomes more important when associated with smoking, hypertension and diabetes. There is also an important interaction with age. In men, there is a doubling of risk from serum cholesterol in the lowest population quintile (<200 mg/dl; 5.2 mmol/l) to the highest (>260 mg/dl; >6.7 mmol/l).

Hypertension

Both diastolic and systolic hypertension have been shown to be risk factors for myocardial infarction and cardiovascular death. The relative risk of persistently elevated blood pressure of >160 mmHg systolic is 4 times the risk compared with systolic blood pressure of <120 mmHg.

The relative risk of persistently elevated diastolic blood pressure >100 mmHg is 3 times higher when compared with a diastolic pressure of <80 mmHg. Research data have shown that reduction in diastolic pressure of 5–6 mmHg and systolic pressure of 10–14 mmHg over 5 years with drug therapy does reduce cardiac mortality and non-fatal myocardial infarction in elderly people by about 20%, and in younger people by about 14%. Data from the longitudinal epidemiological study in Framingham showed that left ventricular hypertrophy diagnosed by echocardiography is associated with a twofold increased risk in death in women and a 1.5-fold increased risk in men over a 4-year period.

Diabetes mellitus

This is a major risk factor for premature vascular disease, stroke, myocardial infarction and death. Diabetes increases the risk of developing coronary heart disease by 1.5 times at age 40–49 and by 1.7 times at age 50–59 in men and by 3.7 times at age 40–49, and 2.4 times at age 50–59 in women. There are data that show that diabetic control is important for cardiovascular risk, with correlations between cardiovascular events, ischaemic heart disease and death rate and glycosylated haemoglobin. Much more effective risk reduction is associated with aggressive treatment of the commonly associated hypertension, lipid abnormalities and obesity in the diabetic patient.

Obesity

Obesity has been increasing in epidemic proportions and confers a prognostic disadvantage. Those with body mass index (weight/ht^2) of 25–29 kg/m^2 are considered to be overweight and those >32 are classified as obese. The latter have a twofold relative increase in mortality from all causes and a threefold increase in cardiovascular death. One study showed that a high body mass index was associated with an increase risk of death per se, especially when it was present in young people aged 30–44 years. More recent evidence suggests that waist circumference is an important independent risk factor as truncal or visceral obesity appears to be more atherogenic. An expanded waist circumference is a necessary criterion for the diagnosis of the metabolic syndrome, in addition to at least two of the other four criteria (Table 1.2).

Table 1.2 International Diabetes Federation definition of metabolic syndrome – focus on waist circumference.

Abdominal obesity plus at least two of the following:	>94 cm male, >80 cm female
Elevated triglycerides	≥1.7 mmol/l
Reduced HDL-cholesterol	<1.0 mmol/l male, 1.3 mmol/l female
Raised blood pressure	>130/80 mmHg
Raised fasting plasma glucose	≥5.6 mmol/l

HDL, High-density lipoprotein.

Despite the presence of the *obesity paradox* – overweight and obese patients with established cardiovascular disease seem to have a more favourable prognosis than leaner patients – there is data to support purposeful weight reduction in the prevention and treatment of cardiovascular diseases. Furthermore, interventional trials involving bariatric surgery for severe obesity have shown that significant weight reduction resulted in significantly reduced mortality.

Physical activity and fitness

There is a close inverse relationship between cardiorespiratory fitness and cardiac outcomes such as coronary disease and death. This can be readily assessed by exercise tolerance testing. Patients with a low level of cardiorespiratory fitness have a 70% higher risk for all-cause mortality and a 56% higher risk for coronary or cardiovascular events compared with those with a high level of fitness. Those with intermediate levels of fitness have a 40% higher mortality risk and a 47% higher coronary or cardiovascular event rate than those with higher fitness. Following acute myocardial infarction or coronary artery bypass graft (CABG), cardiac rehabilitation programmes that promote exercise and weight loss can improve cardiometabolic risk profiles of patients.

Gender

Men have twice the cardiovascular mortality as women at all ages and in all parts of the world. This was thought to be related to the beneficial effect of female sex hormones, especially oestrogens, as the cardiovascular risk in women increases after the menopause. However, two large randomised controlled trials showed that hormone replacement therapy (HRT) did not reduce the cardiovascular risk in women; rather, the thrombotic effects of oestrogens precipitated fatal and non-fatal cardiovascular events, especially in the early years of treatment. Women appear to possess differently weighted risk factors than men for reasons that are unclear.

More recent data have shown strong associations of accelerated atherosclerosis with low levels of testosterone in men followed up for 4–8 years. Low testosterone level in men has been shown to be linked with increased mortality. Male HRT has not yet been shown to reduce cardiovascular risk, although results from animal studies are encouraging.

Psychosocial factors

Some psychosocial factors double the risk of developing cardiovascular disease. Social class has an important effect on mortality from heart disease with people in low-income groups having an excess mortality compared with high-income earners. This is not simply related to deprivation. Within the same working cohort (e.g. Whitehall civil servants), cardiovascular events and mortality were found to be 2–3 times higher in those workers with low socioeconomic status compared with those with high socioeconomic status. In fact, there is little relationship between actual average income and life expectancy. It is not just a matter of money. Mortality is 2–3 times higher in people with poor social links than in those with good social support networks. The reasons are unclear but they are not explained by differences in other known risk factors such as smoking.

Depression

Depression carries an adverse prognosis, especially in association with coronary artery disease and is associated with an eightfold increase in cardiovascular death. Patients with depression have a fivefold increased mortality after acute myocardial infarction. There are no data to suggest that treatment of depression with any specific therapy reverses the excess mortality. Depression also influences the outcome after coronary artery bypass surgery. After controlling for age, sex, number of grafts, diabetes, smoking, left ventricular ejection fraction and previous myocardial infarction, moderate or severe depression at the time of surgery increased the risk of death by 2.4 times, and mild to moderate depression that persisted for 6 months conferred a 2.2 times increased risk of death, during a 5-year follow-up period.

How to assess cardiovascular risk

Cardiovascular risk stratification is carried out through clinical history, physical examination and serum biomarkers. Following extensive validation, tools such as the Framingham or Reynolds risk scores have been adopted in clinical practice by most primary care practitioners. These scores can identify patients with established risk factors who are at greater risk and would most likely benefit from primary prevention. There are also a number of risk estimates that can be provided electronically from the internet (www.riskscore.org.uk; www.bhsoc.org) that have used large populations on which to base risk assessment. They may have some limitations as they are spot estimates that are critically dependent on age as well as actual measurements of blood pressure and cholesterol – which can fluctuate.

More recently, non-invasive imaging of coronary plaque using cardiac magnetic resonance (CMR) and calcification with measurement of coronary calcium using multislice computed tomography (MSCT) scanning have also been used to identify higher risk populations. However, it is as yet uncertain whether treatment modification in this group will result in improved clinical outcome.

Effects of drug treatments

There are two distinct groups of patients who are treated with drug therapy. The first includes those with risk factors for the development of premature vascular disease who do not as yet have overt disease, and is categorised as *primary prevention*. The second includes those patients who have overt cardiovascular disease, such as previous myocardial infarction, peripheral vascular disease and stroke, and is categorised as *secondary prevention*. The physician must weigh up the risks and benefits of treatment in each individual patient. For example, in patients with overt vascular disease the threshold for drug treatment is much lower because there is a higher benefit to risk ratio from the known drug treatment. In those patients who are at risk but who do not yet have overt disease, the risks may outweigh the benefits especially if the overall likelihood of a cardiovascular event is small. Age has a large effect here as the risk of developing vascular disease increases exponentially over the age of 65. Moreover, the absolute risk of an event increases with age, so decisions about the appropriateness of primary prevention need to be reviewed on a regular basis as the patient ages. There are risk calculators available to help the physician make treatment decisions.

Aspirin

Aspirin reduces platelet activation by the inhibition of cyclooxygenase-1 (COX-1) enzyme in platelets, blocking the synthesis of prostaglandin G2/H2 and thromboxane A_2. It is the most commonly prescribed drug for the prevention of atherothrombotic events. Its use in patients early after acute myocardial infarction is associated with a reduction in mortality of about 25% (ISIS-2 study). When used in patients with chronic stable angina, there is some evidence that myocardial infarction and sudden death as a combined end point is reduced by about 30%. The benefit is seen almost immediately on starting the drug. However, the benefit of aspirin is to postpone events and not to prevent them. By comparing the event rate in patients taking aspirin and placebo, it is possible to estimate the delay in events conferred by the drug. The average benefit is a delay in event rate of maximum 24 months with aspirin. Aspirin for primary prevention remains controversial as the relatively small benefit is offset by gastrointestinal problems such as bleeding.

Clopidogrel

A thienopyridine derivative, clopidogrel prevents adenosine diphosphate (ADP)-mediated activation of platelets, thereby blocking activation of the glycoprotein IIb/IIIa complex.

In terms of primary prevention, clopidogrel offers no benefit over aspirin and may even cause harm. In the CHARISMA study, a long-term trial of aspirin combined with clopidogrel versus aspirin alone, there was no significant benefit over aspirin alone and a suggestion of harm in those patients who had risk factors for cardiovascular disease compared with those who had overt disease. However, in patients with overt vascular disease, the drug has been shown to reduce cardiovascular events by about the same degree as aspirin.

In the setting of acute non-ST segment elevation acute coronary syndome, patients had fewer ischaemic end points when treated with the combination of clopidogrel and aspirin compared with aspirin alone, irrespective of whether percutaneous coronary intervention

(PCI) was performed or not (CURE study). In the setting of acute ST segment myocardial infarction treated with aspirin and thrombolytic therapy, the addition of clopidogrel for 1 month conferred a small but significant benefit at 1 month (CLARITY and COMMIT studies).

Cholesterol-lowering drugs

Statins (3-hydroxy-3-methylglutaryl-coenzyme A (HMG CoA) inhibitors) have been shown to reduce all-cause mortality and cardiovascular events (acute myocardial infarction, angina, stroke) in both primary and secondary prevention of cardiovascular disease (Figure 1.3).

In a meta-analysis involving over 70,000 patients without established cardiovascular disease but with cardiovascular risk factors, statin therapy was associated with a significant risk reduction in all-cause mortality of 12%, in major coronary events of 30% and in major cerebrovascular events of 19%. Moreover, statin use was not associated with an increased risk of cancer.

Statins may have additional antiplatelet and anti-inflammatory benefits. Recently, the JUPITER study showed that rosuvastatin significantly reduced the incidence of major cardiovascular events in apparently healthy people without hyperlipidaemia, but elevated high-sensitivity C-reactive protein (hs-CRP). The proposal that an elevated hs-CRP may be a risk marker or risk factor remains uncertain. Statins have no proven benefit in patients with heart failure.

For patients with clinical evidence of cardiovascular disease (previous myocardial infarction or stroke), large-scale trials have indicated that the baseline annual risk of death is about 3%, which is reduced to 2.5% by taking simvastatin. Similarly, long-term registry studies of patients after coronary bypass surgery have shown that average (50%) survival is about 17 years, which is almost 3% per year. In these registry studies, it is also clear that other factors impact on survival after an event – especially the degree of left ventricular damage and the burden of coronary artery disease (number of diseased vessels). Similarly co-morbidity relating to disease in other organ systems adversely affects survival – especially the presence of diabetes and chronic renal dysfunction.

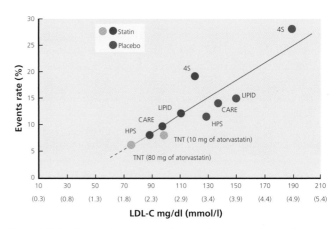

Figure 1.3 Cardiovascular event rates in secondary prevention studies. LIPID, Long-term intervention with pravastatin in ischaemic disease; 4S, Scandinavian simvastatin survival study; CARE, cholesterol and recurrent events; HPS, heart protection study; TNT, treating to new targets; LDL-C, low-density lipoprotein cholesterol.

Supplemental treatment with *n*-3 polyunsaturated fatty acids has also been shown to reduce mortality in patients after acute myocardial infarction, although the effect was small and only 5% of this study population were taking statins at baseline.

β-Adrenoceptor blocking drugs

These drugs reduce mortality by about 10–15% at the time of acute myocardial infarction and have also been shown to reduce late mortality after myocardial infarction by about 20–25%. However, in the setting of chronic stable angina there is no evidence that β-blockers reduce the incidence of myocardial infarction or prolong survival.

Angiotensin-converting enzyme (ACE) inhibitors

These drugs have proven benefit in reducing cardiovascular death both in heart failure and following acute myocardial infarction. In patients with stable coronary disease but without heart failure or left ventricular dysfunction, HOPE and EUROPA studies have shown that patients could gain additional cardiovascular protection with an angiotensin-converting enzyme (ACE) inhibitor. However, in the PEACE study, trandolapril failed to provide any further benefit in terms of death from cardiovascular causes, myocardial infarction or coronary revascularisation. These negative results could be explained by the fact that the study did not include patients with diabetes or high cardiovascular risk, 70% of patients were taking lipid-lowering therapies, more than 90% were treated with aspirin and many patients had undergone prior revascularisation. In a subsequent meta-analysis of these and other studies, ACE inhibitors conferred a significant benefit in reducing mortality, myocardial infarction, stroke and revascularisation. It is therefore currently recommended that ACE inhibitors should be considered for all patients with coronary artery disease. However, this is optional in lower risk patients in whom cardiovascular risk factors are well controlled and revascularisation has been performed.

There are data to show that hypertensive patients treated with ACE inhibitors develop atrial fibrillation less frequently compared with those taking other anti-hypertensive drugs including β-blockers, for example.

Effects of coronary artery revascularisation

In patients with chronic stable angina, CABG surgery may improve prognosis in some subgroups of patients, when compared to medical therapy. However, the benefit of this treatment is small. Evidence from rather dated randomised controlled trials of surgery versus medical treatment has shown the following:

- *Patients with significant left main stem stenosis*: Survival over a 10-year period was increased by an average of 19 months.
- *Patients with significant stenoses of three vessels*: Survival was extended by <6 months.
- *Patients with single or two significant coronary artery stenosis*: Survival was extended by only 1 month.
- *Patients with impairment of left ventricular function*: Survival was extended for about 8 months longer after surgery.

The recent SYNTAX trial of patients with severe coronary artery disease (including severe left main stem disease) showed that at 1 year, CABG was superior to PCI in terms of composite outcome of death, myocardial infarction, stroke and repeat interventions. Repeat revascularisation was significantly higher in the PCI group, and most of these patients were treated with PCI rather than CABG. However, mortality per se was similar in both groups (4.4% PCI vs 3.5% CABG) and the stroke rate was nearly 4 times higher in the CABG group (2.2% vs 0.6% PCI). Longer term follow-up may further clarify the relative benefits of these two procedures.

In patients with acute coronary syndromes (unstable angina, non-ST segment elevation myocardial infarction and ST segment elevation myocardial infarction), the combined end point of myocardial infarction and mortality is reduced by timely intervention by either early PCI or CABG. A review of the clinical trial evidence shows that those patients at highest risk benefit most. In the setting of acute ST segment elevation myocardial infarction, a meta-analysis has shown that primary PCI confers significant mortality and recurrent myocardial infarction benefits.

Conclusion

Although cardiovascular disease continues to exert major socio-economic consequences, there has been a substantive fall in death rates from coronary heart disease over the past decades. Recent evidence highlights the crucial impact of risk factor modification by way of primary and secondary prevention, revascularisation strategies, as well as the modern care of acute coronary syndromes, which incorporates early PCI/CABG policies. The dividing wall between secondary and primary prevention appears to be less significant than before as emerging data highlights the trend towards multiple risk factor modification for all groups. As lowering all risk factors simultaneously has a multiplicative effect in reducing risk, some groups are exploring the interesting potential of a single daily, multi-drug tablet (referred to as the *polypill*). This will include aspirin and a lower dose statin, an ACE inhibitor and a β-blocker for all those above 55 years, diabetics above 35 years and any ages in those with known coronary artery or cerebrovascular disease.

Further reading

Baigent C, Keech A, Kearney PM *et al*. Efficacy and safety of cholesterol-lowering treatment: prospective meta-analysis of data from 90,056 participants in 14 randomised trials of statins. *Lancet* 2005;**366**: 1267–78.

Brugts JJ, Yetgin T, Hoeks SE *et al*. The benefits of statins in people without established cardiovascular disease but with cardiovascular risk factors: meta-analysis of randomised controlled trials. *Br Med J* 2009;**338**:b2376.

Channer KS, Jones TH. Cardiovascular effects of testosterone – implications for the "male menopause". *Heart* 2003;**89**:121–2.

Danchin N, Cucherat M, Thuillez C *et al*. Angiotensin-converting enzyme inhibitors in patients with coronary artery disease and absence of heart failure or left ventricular systolic dysfunction. An overview of long-term randomized controlled trials. *Arch Intern Med* 2006;**166**:787–96.

Kodama S, Saito K, Tanaka S *et al*. Cardiorespiratory fitness as a quantitative predictor of all-cause mortality and cardiovascular events in healthy men and women. *J Am Med Assoc* 2009;**301**:2024–35.

Lavie CJ, Milani RV, Ventura HO. Obesity and cardiovascular disease. Risk factor, paradox, and impact of weight loss. *J Am Coll Cardiol* 2009;**53**: 1925–32.

Lewington S, Whitlock G, Clarke R *et al*. Blood cholesterol and vascular mortality by age, sex and blood pressure: a meta-analysis of individual data from 61 prospective studies with 55,000 vascular deaths. *Lancet* 2007;**370**: 1829–39.

Sjöström L, Narbro K, Sjöström CD *et al*. Effects of bariatric surgery on mortality in Swedish obese subjects. *N Engl J Med* 2007;**357**:741–52.

Smith SC, Allen J, Blair SN *et al*. AHA/ACC guidelines for secondary prevention for patients with coronary and other atherosclerotic vascular disease: 2006 update. *J Am Coll Cardiol* 2006;**47**:2130–9.

Yusuf S, Hawken S, Ounpuu S *et al*. Effect of potentially modifiable risk factors associated with myocardial infarction in 52 countries (the INTERHEART study): case control study. *Lancet* 2004;**364**:937–52.

CHAPTER 2

Pathophysiology and Investigation of Coronary Artery Disease

Ever D. Grech

South Yorkshire Cardiothoracic Centre, Northern General Hospital, Sheffield, UK

OVERVIEW

- Coronary artery disease is the leading cause of death in affluent societies and is usually caused by atheroma causing stenosis or total occlusion
- All patients with definite or possible angina should be referred to a cardiologist where possible
- Effective lifestyle and risk factor modification, as well as optimisation of medical therapy are important general practitioner (GP) roles
- Non-invasive and invasive investigations aim to confirm the diagnosis of angina, provide risk stratification and guide suitability for revascularisation (Figure 2.1)

Pathophysiology

Coronary artery disease is almost always due to atheromatous narrowing and subsequent occlusion of the vessel (Figure 2.2). Early atheroma – from the Greek *athera* (porridge) and *oma* (lump) – may be present from young adulthood onwards. A mature plaque is composed of two constituents, each associated with a particular cell population. The lipid core is mainly released from necrotic 'foam cells' – monocyte-derived macrophages – which migrate into the intima and ingest lipids. The connective tissue matrix is derived from smooth muscle cells, which migrate from the media into the intima, where they proliferate and change their phenotype to form a fibrous capsule around the lipid core (Figure 2.3).

When a plaque produces a >50% diameter stenosis (or >75% reduction in cross-sectional area), reduced blood flow through the coronary artery during exertion may lead to ischaemia and anginal symptoms. The degree of angina may vary considerably between individuals.

Acute coronary events usually arise when thrombus formation follows disruption of a plaque. Intimal injury causes denudation of the thrombogenic matrix or lipid pool and triggers thrombus formation causing subtotal occlusion of the artery, which may precipitate unstable angina. Downstream embolism of this thrombus may produce microinfarcts, resulting in acute non-ST segment elevation myocardial infarction. In acute ST segment elevation myocardial infarction, occlusion is more complete.

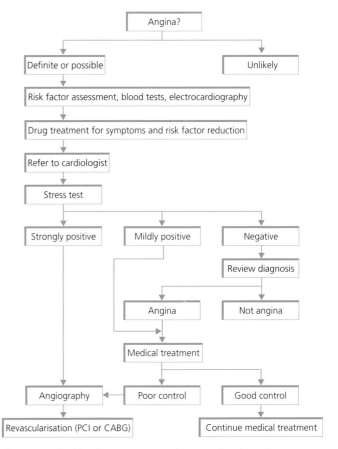

Figure 2.1 Algorithm for management of suspected angina. PCI, percutaneous coronary intervention; CABG, coronary artery bypass grafting.

Investigations

Patients presenting with chest pain may be identified as having definite or possible angina from their history alone. In the former group, risk factor assessment should be undertaken, both to guide diagnosis and because modification of some associated risk factors can reduce cardiovascular events and mortality. A blood count, biochemical screen and thyroid function tests may identify extra factors underlying the onset of angina. Initial drug treatment should include aspirin, a β-blocker and a nitrate. Anti-hypertensive and lipid-lowering drugs may also be given, in conjunction with advice on lifestyle and risk factor modification.

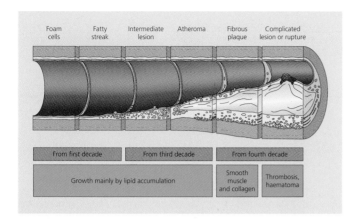

Figure 2.2 Progression of atheromatous plaque from initial lesion to complex and ruptured plaque.

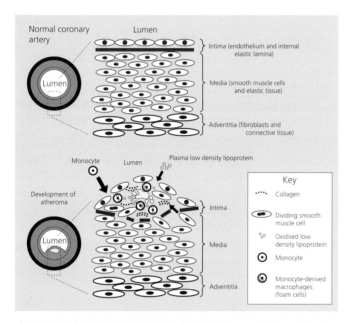

Figure 2.3 Schematic representation of normal coronary artery wall (top) and development of atheroma (bottom).

All patients should be referred to a cardiologist to clarify the diagnosis, optimise drug treatment and assess the need and suitability for revascularisation (which can improve both symptoms and prognosis). Patients should be advised to seek urgent medical help if their symptoms occur at rest or on minimal exertion and if they persist for more than 10 minutes after sublingual nitrate has been taken, as these may herald the onset of an acute coronary syndrome (Table 2.1).

Table 2.1 Priorities for cardiology referral.

Recent onset of symptoms
Rapidly progressive symptoms
Possible aortic stenosis
Severe symptoms (minimal exertion or nocturnal angina)
Angina refractory to medical treatment
Threatened employment

Non-invasive investigations

Electrocardiography
An abnormal electrocardiogram increases the suspicion of significant coronary disease, but a normal result does not exclude it.

Chest X-ray
Patients with angina and no prior history of cardiac disease usually have a normal chest X-ray.

Exercise electrocardiography
This is the most widely used test in evaluating patients with suspected angina (Table 2.2). It is generally safe (risk ratio of major adverse events is 1 in 2500, and of mortality is 1 in 10 000) and provides diagnostic as well as prognostic information. The average sensitivity and specificity is 75%. The test is interpreted in terms of achieved workload, symptoms and electrocardiographic response. A 1-mm depression in the horizontal ST segment is the usual cut-off point for significant ischaemia (Figure 2.4). Poor exercise capacity, an abnormal blood pressure response and profound ischaemic electrocardiographic changes are associated with poor prognosis (Table 2.3a and 2.3b).

Stress echocardiography
Stress-induced impairment of myocardial contraction is a sensitive marker of ischaemia and precedes electrocardiographic changes and angina. Cross-sectional echocardiography can be used to evaluate regional and global left ventricular impairment during ischaemia, which can be induced by exercise or an intravenous infusion of drugs that increase myocardial contraction and heart rate (such as dobutamine) or dilate coronary arterioles (such as dipyridamole or adenosine). The test has a higher sensitivity and specificity than exercise electrocardiography and is useful in patients whose physical condition limits exercise.

Table 2.2 Exercise stress testing.

Indications	Contraindications
Confirmation of suspected angina	Acute cardiac failure
Evaluation of extent of myocardial ischaemia and prognosis	Any feverish illness
Risk stratification after myocardial infarction	Left ventricular outflow tract obstruction or hypertrophic cardiomyopathy
Detection of exercise-induced symptoms (such as arrhythmias or syncope)	Severe aortic or mitral stenosis
Evaluation of outcome of interventions (such as PCI or CABG)	Uncontrolled hypertension
Assessment of cardiac transplant	Pulmonary hypertension
Rehabilitation and patient motivation	Recent myocardial infarction
	Severe tachyarrhythmias
	Dissecting aortic aneurysm
	Left main stem stenosis or equivalent
	Complete heart block (in adults)

PCI, percutaneous coronary interventions; CABG, coronary artery bypass graft.

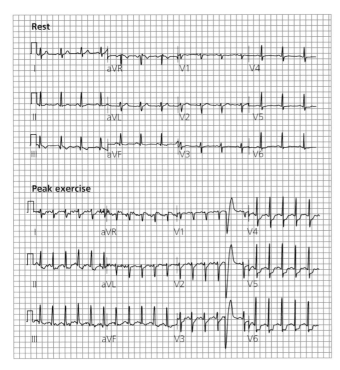

Figure 2.4 Example of strongly positive exercise stress test. After only 2 minutes and 24 seconds of exercise (according to Bruce protocol), the patient developed chest pain and electrocardiography showed marked ischaemic changes (maximum 3-mm ST segment depression in lead V6).

Table 2.3a Main end points for exercise electrocardiography.

Target heart rate achieved (>85% of maximum predicted heart rate)
ST segment depression >1 mm (downsloping or planar depression of greater predictive value than upsloping depression)
Slow ST recovery to normal (>5 min)
Decrease in systolic blood pressure >20 mmHg
Increase in diastolic blood pressure >15 mmHg
Progressive ST segment elevation or depression
ST segment depression >3 mm without pain
Arrhythmias (atrial fibrillation, ventricular tachycardia)

Table 2.3b Features indicative of a strongly positive exercise test.

Exercise limited by angina to <6 min of Bruce protocol
Failure of systolic blood pressure to increase >10 mmHg, or fall with evidence of ischaemia
Widespread marked ST segment depression >3 mm
Prolonged recovery time of ST changes (>6 min)
Development of ventricular tachycardia
ST elevation in the absence of prior myocardial infarction

Radionuclide myocardial perfusion imaging

Thallium-201 or technetium-99m (^{99m}Tc-sestamibi, ^{99m}Tc-tetrofosmin) is injected intravenously at peak stress, and its myocardial distribution relates to coronary flow. Images are acquired with a gamma camera (Figure 2.5). This test can distinguish between reversible and irreversible ischaemia (the latter signifying infarcted tissue). Although it is expensive and requires specialised equipment, it is useful in patients whose exercise test is non-diagnostic or whose exercise ability is limited.

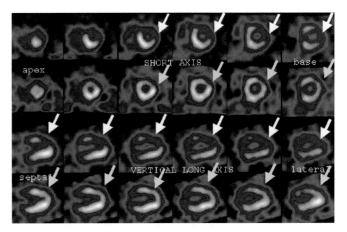

Figure 2.5 Tc^{99m} (tetrafosmin) perfusion scan showing reversible antero-lateral wall ischaemia, induced by intravenous dobutamine infusion (white arrows). Normal rest images are shown (yellow arrows).

A multigated acquisition (MUGA) scan assesses left ventricular function and can reveal salvageable myocardium in patients with chronic coronary artery disease. It can be performed with either thallium scintigraphy at rest or metabolic imaging with fluorodeoxyglucose by means of either positron emission tomography (PET) or single photon emission computed tomography (SPECT).

Cardiac magnetic resonance imaging (MRI)

Magnetic resonance imaging (MRI) is an imaging technique that uses a magnetic field and radio waves to image the body, and X-ray radiation is not required. It has emerged as an important modality to assess cardiac structure, wall motion and perfusion imaging. It is also able to differentiate viable myocardium from infarcted tissue, which may guide revascularisation strategy (Figure 2.6). Stress MRI may offer an alternative to SPECT and stress echocardiography in the functional evaluation of coronary artery disease.

Cardiac multidetector computed tomography (MDCT)

Recent advances in multidetector computed tomography (MDCT) allow sufficient spatial resolution for direct non-invasive coronary artery imaging and has reasonably good diagnostic accuracy for detection of significant lesions in large coronary arteries. It is particularly useful in evaluating the origin, course and patency of anomalous coronary arteries and grafts (Figure 2.7). It may also detect calcium within an atheromatous plaque and has been used in 'calcium scoring', which may indicate the presence of significant coronary artery disease. Calcium scoring is probably best used as a risk factor rather than as a diagnostic test.

Invasive investigations

Coronary angiography

The only absolute way to evaluate coronary artery disease is by angiography (Figure 2.8, Table 2.4). However, as the initial response to atherosclerosis is a compensatory dilatation of the coronary

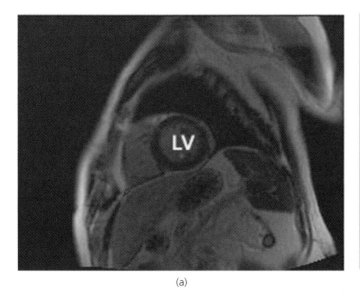

(a)

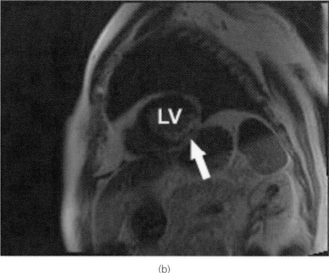

(b)

Figure 2.6 (a) Cardiac magnetic resonance image of a normal heart showing circular LV in a short axis view. (b) Inferior and inferolateral LV scarring due to right coronary artery occlusion. Contrast enhancement of the infarcted myocardium is seen (arrow) following intravenous administration of a gadolinium chelate, which diffuses into interstitium (infarcted myocardium) but not myocardial cells. The increased concentration of gadolinium in infarcted myocardium results in hyper-enhancement. LV, left ventricle.

Table 2.4 Main indications for coronary angiography.

Uncertain diagnosis of angina (coronary artery disease cannot be excluded by non-invasive testing)

Assessment of feasibility and appropriateness of various forms of treatment (percutaneous intervention, bypass surgery, medical)

Class I or II stable angina with positive stress test or class III or IV angina without positive stress test

Angina not controlled by drug treatment

Unstable angina or non-ST segment elevation myocardial infarction (higher risk patients)

Acute ST segment elevation myocardial infarction – including cardiogenic shock, ineligibility for thrombolytic treatment, failed thrombolytic reperfusion, reinfarction or positive stress test

Life-threatening ventricular arrhythmia

Angina after bypass surgery or percutaneous intervention

Before valve surgery or corrective heart surgery to assess occult coronary artery disease

artery, angiography may underestimate the degree of generalised atherosclerosis.

It is usually performed as part of cardiac catheterisation, which includes left ventricular angiography and haemodynamic measurements, providing a more complete evaluation of an individual's cardiac status. Cardiac catheterisation is safely performed as a day case procedure.

Patients must be fully informed of the purpose of the procedure as well as its risks and limitations. Major complications, though rare in experienced hands, include death (risk ratio 1 in 1500), stroke (1 in 1000), coronary artery dissection (1 in 1000) and arterial access complications (1 in 500). Risks depend on the individual patient, and predictors include age, coronary anatomy (such as severe left main stem disease), impaired left ventricular function, valvar heart disease, the clinical setting and non-cardiac disease. The commonest complications are transient or minor and include arterial access

bleeding and haematoma, pseudoaneurysm, arrhythmias, reactions to the contrast medium and vagal reactions (during sheath insertion or removal).

Before the procedure, patients usually fast and may be given a sedative. Although a local anaesthetic is used, arterial access (femoral, brachial or radial) may be mildly uncomfortable. Patients do not usually feel the catheters once they are inside the arteries. Transient angina may occur during injection of contrast medium, usually because of a severely diseased artery. Patients should be warned that, during left ventricular angiography, the large volume of contrast medium may cause a transient hot flush and a strange awareness of urinary incontinence (and can be reassured that this does not actually happen). Modern contrast agents rarely cause nausea and vomiting.

Insertion of an arterial sheath with a haemostatic valve minimises blood loss and allows catheter exchange. Three types of catheter, which come in a variety of shapes and diameters, are commonly used (Figure 2.9). Two have a single hole at the end and are designed to facilitate controlled engagement of the distal tip within the coronary artery ostium. Contrast medium is injected through the lumen of the catheter, and moving X-ray images are obtained and recorded. Other catheters may be used for graft angiography. The 'pigtail' catheter has an end hole and several side holes and is passed across the aortic valve into the left ventricle. It allows injection of 30–40 ml of contrast medium over 3–5 seconds by a motorised pump, providing visualisation of left ventricular contraction over two to four cardiac cycles (Figure 2.10). Aortic and ventricular pressures are also recorded during the procedure.

Intravascular ultrasound (IVUS)

In contrast to angiography, which gives a two-dimensional luminal silhouette with little information about the vessel wall, intravascular

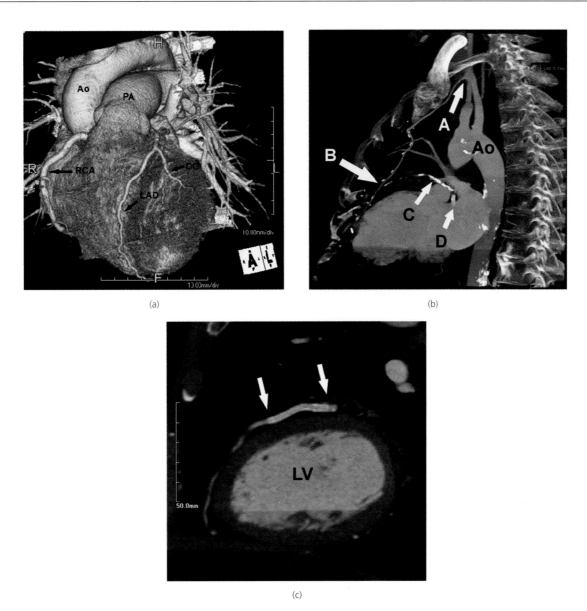

(a)

(b)

(c)

Figure 2.7 (a) Three-dimensional 64-slice cardiac computed tomography scan. (Ao, aorta; PA, pulmonary artery; RCA, right coronary artery; LAD, left anterior descending artery; DG, diagonal artery.) (b) Cardiac computed tomography scan showing course of patent left internal mammary artery (A and B) supplying the native distal LAD artery. The proximal and mid-LAD artery is heavily calcified (C) and there is a visible stent in the left circumflex artery (D). There is also calcification of the aortic arch and descending aorta (Ao). (c) Patent coronary stent (between two arrows) in left anterior descending artery.

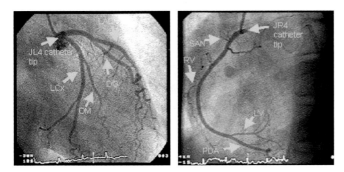

Figure 2.8 Angiogram of normal left and right coronary arteries. LAD, left anterior descending artery; DG, diagonal artery; LCx, left circumflex artery; OM, obtuse marginal artery; SAN, sino-atrial node artery; RV, right ventricular branch artery; LV, left ventricular branch artery; PDA, posterior descending artery; JL4, left 4 Judkins; JR4, right 4 Judkins.

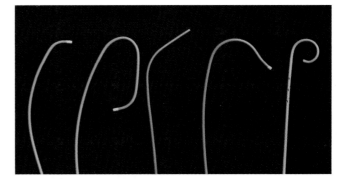

Figure 2.9 Commonly used diagnostic catheters (from left to right): right Judkins, left Judkins, multipurpose, left Amplatz and pigtail.

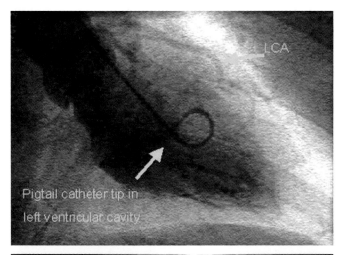

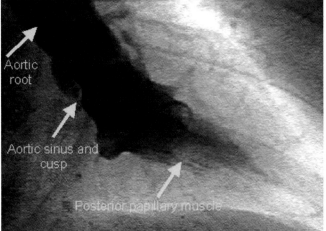

Figure 2.10 Left ventricular angiogram during diastole (top) and systole (bottom), after injection of contrast medium via a pigtail catheter, showing good contractility. LCA, left coronary artery.

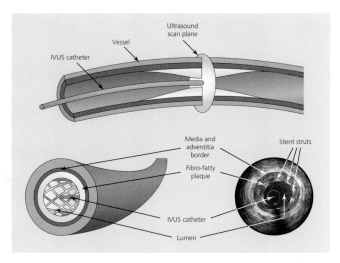

Figure 2.11 The IVUS catheter (above) and images showing a stent in a diseased coronary artery (below). IVUS, intravascular ultrasound.

ultrasound (IVUS) provides a cross-sectional, three-dimensional image of the full circumference of the artery (Figure 2.11). It allows precise measurement of plaque length, thickness and minimum lumen diameter, as well as characterise the plaque's composition. The latter may be colour enhanced to demonstrate a fibrous, fibro-fatty, necrotic core and dense calcium (Figure 2.12).

It is often used to clarify ambiguous angiographic findings and to identify wall dissections or thrombus. It is most useful during percutaneous coronary intervention (PCI), when target lesions can be assessed before, during and after the procedure and at follow-up. The procedure can also show that stents which seem to be well deployed on angiography are, in fact, suboptimally expanded. Its main limitations are the need for an operator experienced in its use and its expense; for these reasons, it is not routinely used in many centres.

Doppler flow wire and pressure wire

Unlike angiography or IVUS, the Doppler flow wire and pressure wire provide information on the physiological importance of a diseased coronary artery. They are usually used when angiography shows a stenosis that is of intermediate severity or to determine the functional severity of a residual stenosis after PCI.

Intracoronary adenosine is used to dilate the distal coronary vessels in order to maximise coronary flow (hyperaemia). The Doppler flow wire has a velocity sensor at its tip, which is positioned beyond the stenosis to measure peak flow velocity. The pressure wire has a pressure transducer which allows recordings of coronary mean arterial pressures distal to the stenosis (Pd), at maximal adenosine hyperaemia. Mean aortic pressure (Pa) is simultaneously measured by the guiding catheter. Myocardial fractional flow reserve (FFR) is derived from the distal/proximal pressure ratio (Pd:Pa). A diagnostic cut-off at 0.75 is independent of blood pressure and heart rate changes, and takes into account the contribution of collateral blood supply. The FAME study randomised 1005 patients with multivessel disease to either angiographically or FFR-guided PCI. Those in the former group underwent PCI if the lesion was >50% and in the latter only if FFR >0.8. After 1 year, FFR-guided PCI reduced the risk of death, myocardial infarction or repeat revascularisation by 30% and death or myocardial infarction by 35%, compared with the practice of using angiography alone to guide stenting decisions. This benefit was maintained after 2 years and this study underlines the potential benefit of the pressure wire.

Optical coherence tomography (OCT)

Optical coherence tomography (OCT) is a recently developed optical imaging technique that uses near-infrared light back-reflection to provide high-resolution (approximately 10 times higher than IVUS) cross-sectional images of coronary arteries. It is useful in determining tissue characterisation of plaques (especially vulnerable thin-capped plaques), intracoronary thrombus, stent expansion and restenosis (Figure 2.13). However, an inherent limitation of OCT is that imaging is only possible by displacement of blood with saline. Future-generation OCT systems may overcome some of the current technical limitations.

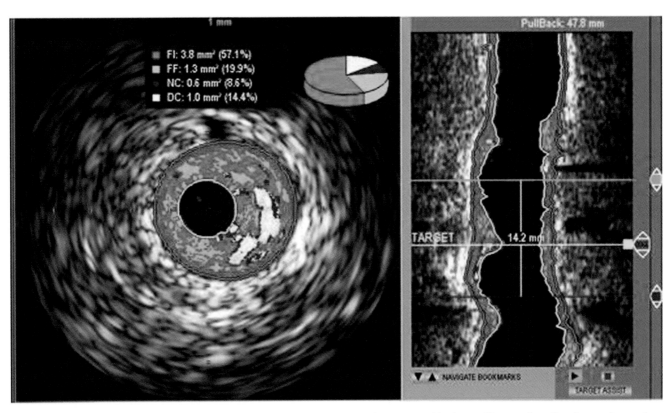

Figure 2.12 Intravascular ultrasound demonstrating colour enhancement according to plaque composition (green, fibrous; yellow, fibro-fatty; red, necrotic core; white, dense calcium).

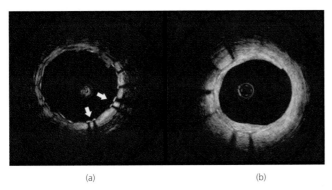

(a)   (b)

Figure 2.13 OCT images of stented coronary artery (a) with well-apposed stent struts (arrows), and at 1 year (b) showing only mild in-stent restenosis due to neointimal coverage.

Angioscopy

This technique, which requires occlusion of coronary blood flow and infusion of saline into the artery, allows direct internal visualisation of the coronary artery by a fibre-optic catheter. Overall image clarity is poor and interpretation can be difficult. In contrast to IVUS or OCT, it gives no quantitative information or detail on plaque morphology and composition. In view of its cost and poor diagnostic yield, it is now rarely used.

Further reading

Mark DB, Shaw L, Harrell FE Jr *et al.* Prognostic value of a treadmill exercise score in outpatients with suspected coronary artery disease. *N Engl J Med* 1991;**325**:849–53.

Marwick TH, Case C, Sawada S *et al.* Prediction of mortality using dobutamine echocardiography. *J Am Coll Cardiol* 2001;**37**:754–60.

Mintz GS, Nissen SE, Anderson WD *et al.* American College of Cardiology clinical expert consensus document on standards for acquisition, measurement and reporting of intravascular ultrasound studies (IVUS). *J Am Coll Cardiol* 2001;**37**:1478–92.

Scanlon PJ, Faxon DP, Audet AM *et al.* ACC/AHA guidelines for coronary angiography. A report of the American College of Cardiology/American Heart Association Task Force on Practice Guidelines (Committee on Coronary Angiography). *J Am Coll Cardiol* 1999;**33**:1756–824.

Tonino PAL, De Bruyne B, Pijls NHJ *et al.* Fractional flow reserve versus angiography for guiding percutaneous coronary intervention *N Engl J Med* 2009;**360**:213–24.

CHAPTER 3

Percutaneous Coronary Intervention (I): History and Development

Ever D. Grech

South Yorkshire Cardiothoracic Centre, Northern General Hospital, Sheffield, UK

OVERVIEW

- Coronary artery bypass graft (CABG) and percutaneous catheter-attached devices are the two major treatments available for myocardial revascularisation

- The first percutaneous transluminal coronary angioplasty (PTCA) was carried out just 33 years ago; considerable improvements in equipment now allow very complex stenotic lesions to be dilated

- PTCA increases luminal area by outward plaque compression, fracturing and fissuring. Such trauma may cause acute closure and severe restenosis

- Intracoronary stents have had a major impact in procedure safety and reduction in restenosis rates. They have become an essential component of coronary intervention and there has been a massive increase in their usage (Table 3.1). Approximately, three percutaneous coronary intervention (PCI) procedures are carried out for every one bypass surgical operation

- Other catheter devices have not been shown to be as practical or as effective as the stent in reducing restenosis

Table 3.1 Canadian Cardiovascular Society classification of angina.

Class I
- No angina during ordinary physical activity such as walking or climbing stairs
- Angina during strenuous, rapid or prolonged exertion

Class II
- Slight limitation of ordinary activity
- Angina on walking or climbing stairs rapidly; walking uphill; walking or climbing stairs shortly after meals, in cold or wind, when under emotional stress or only in the first few hours after waking
- Angina on walking more than two blocks (100–200 m) on the level or climbing more than one flight of stairs at normal pace and in normal conditions

Class III
- Marked limitation of ordinary physical activity
- Angina on walking one or two blocks on the level or climbing one flight of stairs at normal pace and in normal conditions

Class IV
- Inability to carry out any physical activity without discomfort
- Includes angina at rest

The term *angina pectoris* was introduced by Heberden in 1772 to describe a syndrome characterised by a sensation of 'strangling and anxiety' in the chest. Today, it is used for chest discomfort attributed to myocardial ischaemia arising from increased myocardial oxygen consumption. This is often induced by physical exertion, and the commonest aetiology is atheromatous coronary artery disease. The terms *chronic* and *stable* refer to anginal symptoms that have been present for at least several weeks without major deterioration. However, symptom variation occurs for several reasons, such as mental stress, ambient temperature, consumption of alcohol or large meals and factors that may increase coronary tone such as drugs and hormonal change.

Classification

The Canadian Cardiovascular Society has provided a graded classification of angina, which has become widely used (Table 3.1). In clinical practice, it is important to describe accurately specific activities associated with angina in each patient. This should include walking distance, frequency and duration of episodes.

History of myocardial revascularisation

In the management of chronic stable angina, there are two invasive techniques available for myocardial revascularisation: coronary artery bypass surgery and catheter-attached devices. Although coronary artery bypass surgery was introduced in 1968, the first percutaneous transluminal coronary angioplasty (PTCA) was not performed until September 1977 by Andreas Gruentzig, a Swiss radiologist, in Zurich. The patient, 38-year-old Adolph Bachman, underwent successful angioplasty to a proximal left coronary artery lesion and remains well to this day. After the success of the operation, six patients were successfully treated with PTCA in that year.

By today's standards, the early procedures used very cumbersome equipment: guide catheters were large and could easily traumatise the vessel, there were no guidewires and balloon catheters were large with low burst pressures. As a result, the procedure was limited to patients with refractory angina, good left ventricular function and a discrete, proximal, concentric and non-calcific lesion in a single major coronary artery with no involvement of major side branches or angulations. Consequently, it was considered feasible in less than 10% of all patients needing revascularisation.

Developments in percutaneous coronary intervention

During 1977–1986 guide catheters, guidewires and balloon catheter technology were improved, with slimmer profiles and increased tolerance to high inflation pressures (Figure 3.1). With advances in equipment and increased experience, more complex lesions were treated and in more acute situations (Figure 3.2). Consequently, percutaneous coronary intervention (PCI) can now be undertaken in over two-thirds of patients needing revascularisation, and it is also offered to high-risk patients for whom coronary artery bypass surgery may be considered too dangerous.

Although PTCA causes plaque compression, the major change in lumen geometry is caused by fracturing and fissuring of the atheroma, extending into the vessel wall at variable depths and lengths (Figure 3.3). This injury accounts for the two major limitations of PTCA – acute vessel closure and restenosis.

Acute vessel closure – following balloon angioplasty, this usually occurred within the first 24 hours of the procedure in about 3–5% of cases and followed vessel dissection, acute thrombus formation or both. Important clinical consequences included myocardial infarction, emergency coronary artery bypass surgery and death.

Restenosis – the process of renarrowing of a coronary artery lumen, which begins at the time of the procedure and may persist up to the first 6 months after angioplasty. The incidence of restenosis after balloon angioplasty is 25–50% (higher after vein graft angioplasty), which often necessitated further intervention when angina and ischaemia recurred.

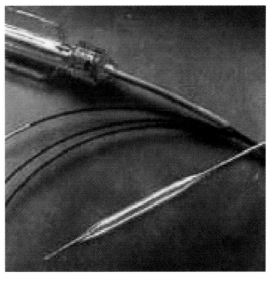

Figure 3.2 Modern balloon catheter: its low profile facilitates lesion crossing, the flexible shaft allows tracking down tortuous vessels and the balloon can be inflated to high pressures without distortion or rupture.

The development of restenosis involves three processes. The first two are mechanical and the third is biological (Figure 3.4).

- *Elastic recoil*, which occurs soon after the procedure is due to the inherent elasticity of the artery.
- *Negative remodelling* may take weeks or months and involves the outermost layer of the artery (adventitia), which shrinks inwards as the vessel begins to heal itself.
- *Neointimal hyperplasia* (often called *neointimal proliferation*) is a biological wound healing response to arterial wall injury. Such injury initiates an inflammatory response leading to neointimal hyperplasia consisting of smooth muscle cell proliferation, migration and production of extracellular matrix (collagen and proteoglycans) (Figure 3.5).

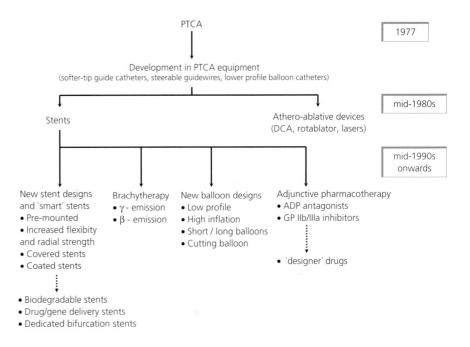

Figure 3.1 Major milestones in percutaneous coronary intervention. PTCA, percutaneous transluminal coronary angioplasty; DCA, directional coronary atherectomy; ADP, adenosine diphosphate; GP IIb/IIIa, glycoprotein IIb/IIIa.

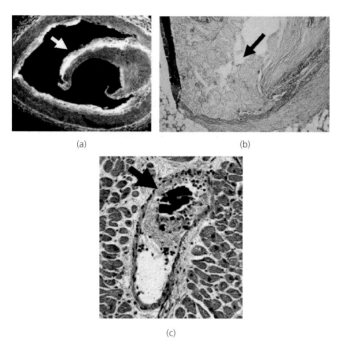

(a)   (b)

(c)

Figure 3.3 Micrographs showing arterial barotrauma caused by coronary angioplasty. (a) Coronary arterial dissection with large flap. (b) Deep fissuring within coronary artery wall atheroma. (c) Fragmented plaque tissue (dark central calcific plaque surrounded by fibrin and platelet-rich thrombus), which may embolise in distal arterioles to cause infarction.

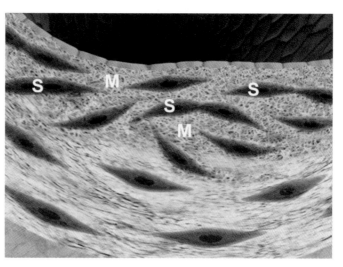

Figure 3.5 Proliferating smooth muscle cells (S), which increase cellular mass in the neointima and extracellular matrix (M) lead to restenosis.

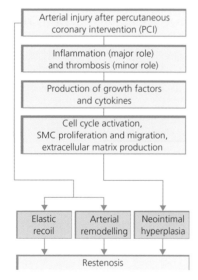

Figure 3.4 Restenosis cascade following coronary angioplasty. SMC, smooth muscle cell.

Diagram contents:
- Arterial injury after percutaneous coronary intervention (PCI)
- Inflammation (major role) and thrombosis (minor role)
- Production of growth factors and cytokines
- Cell cycle activation, SMC proliferation and migration, extracellular matrix production
- Elastic recoil | Arterial remodelling | Neointimal hyperplasia
- Restenosis

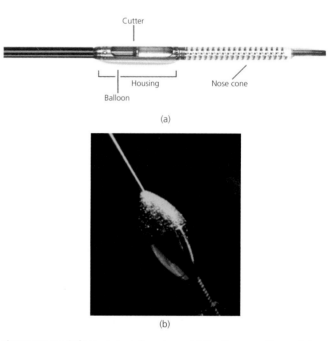

Figure 3.6 Tools for coronary atherectomy. (a) The Simpson atherocath has a cutter in a hollow cylindrical housing. The cutter rotates at 2000 rpm, and excised atheromatous tissue is pushed into the distal nose cone. (b) The Rotablator burr is coated with 10-µm diamond chips to create an abrasive surface. The burr, connected to a drive shaft and a turbine powered by compressed air, rotates at speeds up to 200,000 rpm.

Figure 3.6a labels: Cutter, Housing, Nose cone, Balloon, (a)
Figure 3.6b label: (b)

Drills, cutters and lasers

In the 1980s, two main developments aimed at limiting the problems of acute vessel closure and restenosis emerged. The first were devices to remove plaque material, such as by rotational atherectomy, directional coronary atherectomy, transluminal extraction catheter and excimer laser (Figure 3.6). By avoiding the vessel wall trauma seen during PTCA, it was envisaged that both acute vessel closure and restenosis rates would be reduced.

However, early studies showed that, although acute closure rates were reduced, there was no significant reduction in restenosis. Moreover, these devices were expensive, not particularly user-friendly, and had limited accessibility to more distal stenoses. As a result, they have now become obsolete or niche tools used by relatively few interventionists. They may have an emerging role when used as adjunctive treatment before stenting (especially for large plaques) and in treating diffuse restenosis within a stent.

Intracoronary stents

The second major development was the introduction of intracoronary stents deployed at the site of an atheromatous lesion. These were introduced in 1986 with the objective of tacking down dissection flaps and providing mechanical support. They also markedly reduced elastic recoil and negative remodelling, leading to lower restenosis rates from 30–50% to 15–30%.

The first large randomised studies conclusively showed the superiority of stenting over coronary angioplasty alone, both in clinical and angiographic outcomes, including a significant 30% reduction in restenosis rates. Surprisingly, this was not due to inhibition of neointimal proliferation – in fact, stents may increase this response. The superiority of stenting is that the initial gain in luminal diameter is much greater than after angioplasty alone, mostly because of a reduction in elastic recoil (Table 3.2).

Although neointimal proliferation through the struts of the stent occurs, it is insufficient to cancel out the initial gain, leading to a larger lumen size and hence reduces restenosis. Maximising the vessel lumen is therefore a crucial mechanism for reducing restenosis. 'Bigger is better' is the adage followed in this case (Figure 3.7).

Early stent problems

As a result of initial studies, stents were predominantly used either as 'bail out' devices for acute vessel closure during coronary angioplasty (thus avoiding the need for immediate coronary artery bypass surgery) or for restenosis after angioplasty.

Thrombosis within a stent causing myocardial infarction and death was a major concern, and early aggressive anticoagulation to prevent this led to frequent bleeding complications from arterial puncture wounds as well as major systemic haemorrhage. These problems have now been overcome by the introduction of powerful antiplatelet drugs as a substitute for warfarin.

The risk of thrombosis within a stent diminishes when the stent becomes lined with a new endothelial layer within a few weeks, and hence dual antiplatelet therapy (aspirin and clopidogrel) can be reduced to aspirin alone after the first month. Furthermore, the recognition that suboptimal stent expansion is an important contributor to thrombosis in stents has led to the use of intravascular ultrasound to guide stent deployment and high-pressure inflations to ensure complete stent expansion.

Current practice

A greater understanding of the pathophysiology of stent deployment, combined with the development of more flexible stents (which are pre-mounted on low-profile catheter balloons), has resulted in a massive worldwide increase in stent use, and they have become an essential component of coronary intervention. Low-profile stents have also allowed 'direct' stenting – that is, implanting a stent without the customary balloon pre-dilatation – to become prevalent, with the advantages of economy, shorter procedure time and less radiation from imaging (Figure 3.8).

Most modern stents are expanded by balloon and are made from stainless steel, as well as chromium, platinum, cobalt and other alloys. Their construction and design, metal thickness, surface coverage and radial strength vary considerably.

Stents are now used in most coronary interventions and in a wide variety of clinical settings (Figure 3.9). They substantially increase procedural safety and success, and have markedly reduced the need for emergency coronary artery bypass surgery. Procedures

Table 3.2 Unequivocal indications for use of coronary stents.

- Acute or threatened vessel closure during angioplasty
- Primary reduction in restenosis in de novo lesions in arteries >3.0 mm in diameter
- Focal lesions in saphenous vein grafts
- Recanalised total chronic occlusions
- Primary treatment of acute coronary syndromes

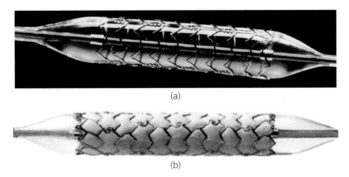

(a)

(b)

Figure 3.7 Coronary stents. (a) Example of intracoronary stent. (b) The coronary stent graft consists of a layer of PTFE (polytetrafluoroethylene) sandwiched between two stents and is useful in sealing perforations, aneurysms and fistulae.

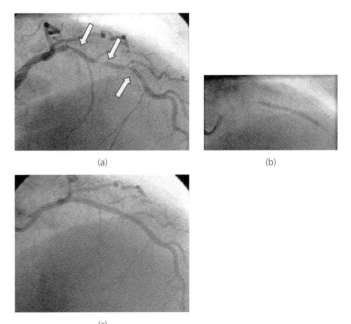

(a)   (b)

(c)

Figure 3.8 Coronary angiogram showing three lesions (arrows) affecting the left anterior descending artery (a). The lesions are stented without pre-dilatation (b), with good results (c).

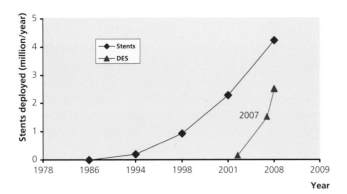

Figure 3.9 Exponential increase in use of intracoronary stents since 1986. In 2008, approximately 4.2 million stents were implanted (four and half times the 1998 rate) and 60% of these were drug-eluting stents (DES).

involving stent deployment are now often referred to as percutaneous coronary interventions (PCI), to distinguish them from conventional balloon angioplasty (PTCA).

A major recent development has been the introduction of drug-eluting stents (also referred to as coated stents), which have further reduced restenosis to very low rates (2–4%). Previously, their high cost limited their use, but with increasing competition among manufacturers, they have become more affordable and now account for approximately 75% of all implanted stents.

Further reading

Costa MA, Foley DP, Serruys PW. Restenosis: the problem and how to deal with it. In: Grech ED, Ramsdale DR, eds. *Practical Interventional Cardiology*. 2nd ed. London: Martin Dunitz, 2002:279–94.

Gruentzig AR. Transluminal dilatation of coronary artery stenosis. *Lancet* 1978;**1**:263.

Meyer BJ, Meer B. Percutaneous transluminal coronary angioplasty of single or multivessel disease and chronic total occlusions. In: Grech ED, Ramsdale DR, eds. *Practical Interventional Cardiology*. 2nd ed. London: Martin Dunitz, 2002:35–54.

Smith SC Jr, Dove JT, Jacobs AK *et al.* ACC/AHA guidelines of percutaneous coronary interventions (revision of the 1993 PTCA guidelines) – executive summary. A report of the American College of Cardiology/American Heart Association Task Force on Practice Guidelines (committee to revise the 1993 guidelines for percutaneous transluminal coronary angioplasty). *J Am Coll Cardiol* 2001;**37**:2215–39.

CHAPTER 4

Percutaneous Coronary Intervention (II): The Procedure

Ever D. Grech

South Yorkshire Cardiothoracic Centre, Northern General Hospital, Sheffield, UK

> **OVERVIEW**
>
> - Relief of anginal symptoms is the principal indication for percutaneous coronary intervention (PCI)
>
> - Although PCI is attractive to patients, its risks, limitations and benefits compared to coronary artery bypass graft (CABG) surgery and medical therapy options must be fully discussed
>
> - PCI complications are significantly lower in centres where large numbers of procedures are carried out by adequately trained and experienced operators
>
> - Restenosis remains an important limitation of PCI, although drug-eluting stents have significantly reduced this problem and have therefore rapidly become the standard of care for the treatment of coronary artery disease

A wide range of patients may be considered for percutaneous coronary intervention (PCI) (Table 4.1). It is essential that the benefits and risks of the procedure, as well as coronary artery bypass graft (CABG) surgery and medical treatment, are discussed with patients (and their families) in detail. They must understand that, although the percutaneous procedure is more attractive than bypass surgery, it has important limitations, including the possibility of restenosis, which may necessitate repeat PCI (or CABG), as well as the potential for incomplete revascularisation compared with surgery. The potential benefits of anti-anginal drug treatment and the need for risk factor modification should also be carefully explained.

Clinical risk assessment

In patients with chronic stable angina, relief of anginal symptoms is the principal clinical indication for percutaneous intervention. We do not know whether the procedure has the same prognostic benefit as bypass surgery although long-term mortality in both groups is broadly similar. Angiographic features determined during initial assessment require careful evaluation to determine the likely success of the procedure and the risk of serious complications.

Until recently, the American College of Cardiology and American Heart Association classified anginal lesions into types

Table 4.1 Clinical indications for percutaneous coronary intervention.

- Chronic stable angina (and positive stress test)
- Objective evidence of ischaemia
- Acute coronary syndrome
- Cardiogenic shock
- After coronary artery bypass surgery (percutaneous intervention to native vessels, arterial or venous conduits)
- Prohibitively high risk for coronary artery bypass surgery
- Elderly patients

(and subtypes) A, B or C based on the severity of lesion characteristics. Because of the ability of stents to overcome many of the complications of percutaneous intervention, this classification has now been superseded by one reflecting low, moderate and high risk (Table 4.2).

Successful percutaneous intervention depends on adequate visualisation of the target stenosis and its adjacent arterial branches. Vessels beyond the stenosis may also be important because of the potential for collateral flow and myocardial support if the target vessel were to occlude abruptly. Factors that adversely affect outcome

Table 4.2 New classification system of stenotic lesions (American College of Cardiology and American Heart Association).

Low risk	Moderate risk	High risk
Discrete (<10 mm)	Tubular (10–20 mm)	Diffuse (>20 mm)
Concentric	Eccentric	–
Readily accessible	Proximal segment moderately tortuous	Proximal segment excessively tortuous
Segment not angular (<45°)	Segment moderately angular (45° – <90°)	Segment extremely angular (≥90°)
Smooth contour	Irregular contour	–
Little or no calcification	Moderate or heavy calcification	
Occlusion not total	Total occlusion <3 months old	Total occlusion >3 months or bridging collateral vessels
Non-ostial	Ostial	–
No major side branch affected	Bifurcated lesions requiring double guidewires	Inability to protect major side branches
No thrombus	Some thrombus	Degenerated vein grafts with friable lesions

---

ABC of Interventional Cardiology, 2nd edition.
© Ever D. Grech. Published 2011 Blackwell Publishing Ltd.

include increasing age, co-morbid disease, pre-existing heart or renal failure, previous myocardial infarction, diabetes, a large area of myocardium at risk, degree of collateralisation, multivessel disease, acute coronary syndrome and in particular cardiogenic shock.

Preparation for intervention

Patients must be fully informed of the purpose of the procedure as well as its risks and limitations before they are asked for their consent. The procedure must always be carried out (or directly supervised) by experienced, high-volume operators (>75 procedures a year) and institutions (>400 a year) (Figure 4.1).

A sedative is often given before the procedure, as well as aspirin and clopidogrel or prasugrel as antiplatelet agents, and the patient's usual anti-anginal drugs. In very high-risk cases, an intra-aortic balloon pump may be used. A prophylactic temporary transvenous pacemaker wire may be inserted in some patients with pre-existing, high-grade conduction abnormality or those at high risk of developing it.

The procedure

For an uncomplicated, single lesion, a percutaneous procedure may take as little as 30 minutes. However, the duration of the procedure and radiation exposure will vary according to the number and complexity of the treated stenoses and vessels.

As with coronary angiography, arterial access (usually femoral but also brachial or radial) under local anaesthesia is required. A guide catheter is introduced and gently engaged at the origin of the coronary artery. The proximal end of the catheter is attached to a Y connector (Figure 4.2). One arm of this connector allows continuous monitoring of arterial blood pressure. Dampening or 'pseudo-ventricularisation' of the arterial tracing may indicate

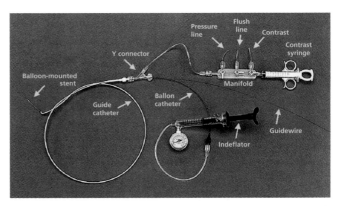

Figure 4.2 Equipment commonly used in percutaneous coronary interventions.

reduced coronary flow because of over-engagement of the guide catheter, catheter tip spasm or a previously unrecognised ostial lesion. The other arm has an adjustable seal, through which the operator can introduce the guidewire and balloon or stent catheter, once the patient has been given heparin as an anticoagulant. A glycoprotein IIb/IIIa inhibitor, which may substantially reduce ischaemic events during PCI, may also be given.

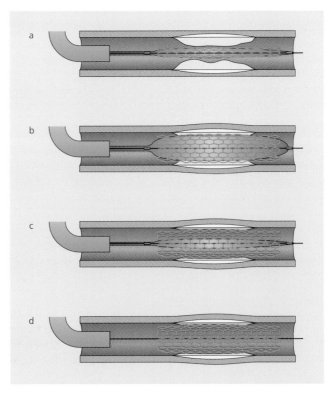

Figure 4.3 Deployment of a balloon-mounted stent across stenotic lesion. Once the guide catheter is satisfactorily engaged, the lesion is crossed with a guidewire and the balloon-mounted stent positioned to cover the lesion (a). It may be necessary to pre-dilate a severe lesion with a balloon to provide adequate passageway for the balloon and stent. The balloon is inflated to expand the stent (b). The balloon is then deflated (c) and withdrawn leaving behind the expanded stent (d), Lastly, the guidewire is removed once the operator is satisfied that a good result has been obtained.

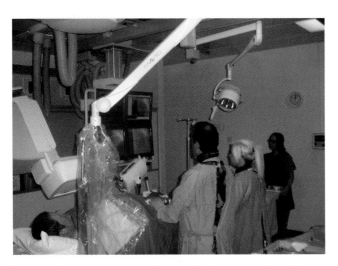

Figure 4.1 Percutaneous coronary intervention in progress. Above the patient's chest is the X-ray imaging camera. Fluoroscopic images, electrocardiogram and haemodynamic data are viewed on eye-level screens. All catheterisation laboratory operators wear lead protection covering body, thyroid and eyes, and there is lead shielding between the primary operator and patient.

Visualised by means of fluoroscopy and intracoronary injections of contrast medium, a soft tipped, steerable guidewire (usually 0.014″ (0.36 mm) diameter) is passed down the coronary artery, across the stenosis, and into a distal branch. A balloon or stent catheter is then passed over the guidewire and positioned at the stenosis (Figure 4.3). The stenosis may then be stented directly or dilated before stenting. Additional balloon dilatation may be necessary after deployment of a stent to ensure its full expansion.

Balloon inflation inevitably stops coronary blood flow, which may induce angina. Patients usually tolerate this quite well, especially if they have been warned beforehand. If it becomes severe or prolonged, however, an intravenous opiate may be given. Ischaemic electrocardiographic changes are often seen at this time, although they are usually transient and return to baseline once the balloon is deflated (usually after 30–60 seconds). During the procedure, it is important to talk to the patient (who may be understandably apprehensive) to let him or her know what is happening, as this encourages a good rapport and co-operation.

Recovery

After the procedure, the patient is transferred to a ward where close monitoring for signs of ischaemia and haemodynamic instability is available. The arterial sheath may be removed when the heparin effect has declined to an acceptable level (according to unit protocols). Femoral arterial sealing devices have some advantages over manual compression: they permit immediate sheath removal and haemostasis, are more comfortable for patients and allow early mobilisation and discharge (Figure 4.4).

After a few hours, the patient should be encouraged to gradually increase mobility, and in uncomplicated cases, discharge is scheduled for the same or the next day. Before discharge, the arterial access site should be examined and the patient advised to seek immediate medical advice if bleeding or chest pain (particularly at rest) occurs. Outpatient follow-up and drug regimens are provided, as well as advice on modification of risk factors and lifestyle.

Complications and sequelae

Complications are substantially lower in centres where large numbers of procedures are carried out by adequately trained and experienced operators. Major complications are uncommon and include death (0.2% but higher in high-risk cases), acute myocardial infarction (1%), which may on rare occasion require emergency coronary artery bypass surgery, embolic stroke (0.5%), cardiac tamponade (0.5%) and major bleeding (1–2%). The latter may be systemic or related to the arterial access site (bleeding, haematoma and pseudoaneurysm).

Minor complications are more common and include allergy to the contrast medium and nephropathy and complications of the access site (bruising/haematomas).

Restenosis within a stent

Compared to balloon angioplasty alone, bare metal stents (BMS) reduce restenosis rates by approximately 30% by preventing elastic

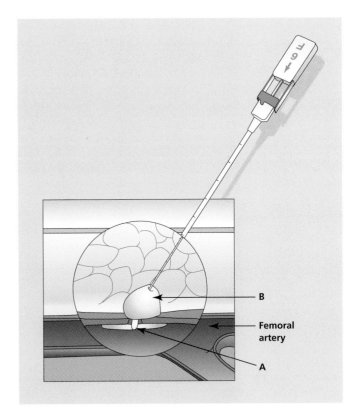

Figure 4.4 Example of a femoral artery closure device. The Angio-Seal device creates a mechanical seal by sandwiching the arteriotomy between an anchor placed against the inner arterial wall (A) and collagen sponge (B), which both dissolve within 60–90 days.

recoil and negative remodelling. However, these stents do not reduce neointimal proliferation and is the most important late sequel of the procedure (Figure 4.5). Restenosis within the stent (known as *in-stent restenosis*) usually develops within 6 months of stenting and has been the Achilles' heel of percutaneous revascularisation. Restenosis is measured in two ways.

Angiographic restenosis

Angiographic restenosis (also referred to as *binary restenosis*) is defined as >50% diameter stenosis at follow-up and is usually assessed by quantitative coronary angiography (QCA). It should be noted that angiographically apparent restenoses do not always lead to recurrent angina (clinical restenosis). In some patients, only mild anginal symptoms recur, and these may be well controlled with anti-anginal drugs, thereby avoiding the need for further intervention.

Restenosis is dependent on several factors. Rates are higher in smaller vessels (Figure 4.6), long and complex stenoses and where there are coexisting conditions such as diabetes. Approximate rates of angiographic restenosis for single lesions are

- 30–50% following balloon angioplasty alone;
- 15–30% following balloon angioplasty and stent;
- 2–4% following balloon angioplasty and drug-eluting stent (DES) (Figure 4.7).

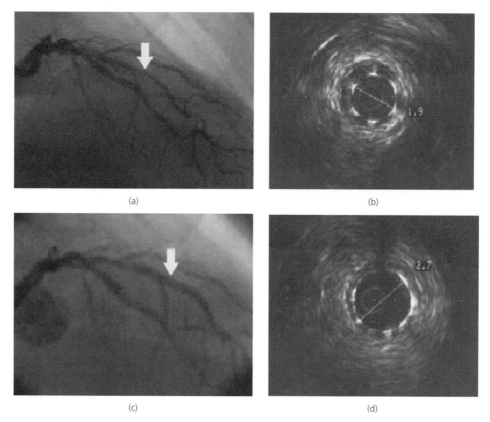

(a)   (b)

(c)   (d)

Figure 4.5 Focal in-stent restenosis. A 2.0-mm stent had been deployed 6 months earlier. After recurrence of angina, angiography showed focal in-stent restenosis (arrow, (a)). This was confirmed with intravascular ultrasound (b), which also revealed that the stent was underexpanded. The stent was further expanded with a balloon catheter, with a good angiographic result (arrow, (c)) and an increased lumen diameter to 2.7 mm (d).

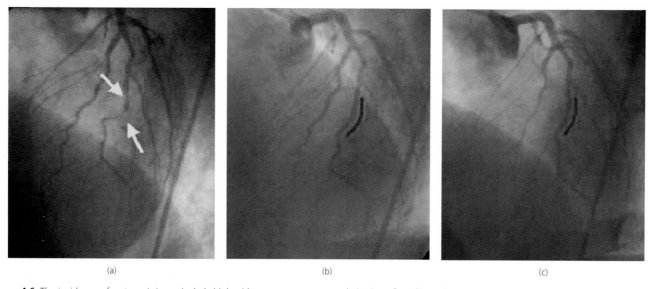

(a)   (b)   (c)

Figure 4.6 The incidence of restenosis is particularly high with percutaneous revascularisation of small vessels. A small diseased diagonal artery (arrows, (a)) in a 58-year old patient with limiting angina was stented with a sirolimus-coated Cypher stent (red line, (b)). After 6 months, no restenosis was present (c), and the patient remained asymptomatic.

Clinical restenosis (with target lesion revascularisation)

Clinical restenosis due to the recurrence of symptoms may necessitate the need for repeat intervention with PCI or CABG – often referred to as *target lesion revascularisation* (TLR). It may occur for reasons other than in-stent restenosis, such as disease progression or a new lesion adjacent to the original treated area (referred to as *target vessel revascularisation*). The TLR rate will typically be about half that of the binary restenosis rate, meaning that binary restenosis can be asymptomatic. Often, an approximate 70% diameter vessel

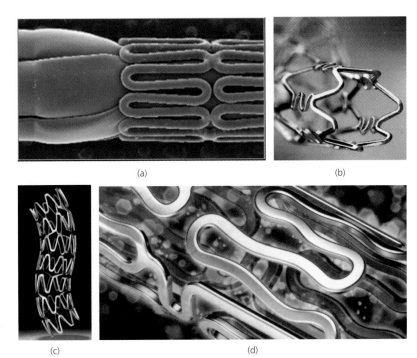

(a)   (b)

(c)   (d)

Figure 4.7 Examples of drug-eluting stents in current use showing differing architecture. Their design allows crimping of the stent on the balloon to a very low profile (a) and maximal flexibility to allow delivery through tortuous vessels and lesions, whilst simultaneously having strong scaffolding properties (radial strength) following deployment.

stenosis is needed for a patient to have ischaemic symptoms. Since binary restenosis is defined as at least a 50% diameter stenosis, there are patients who have binary restenosis but do not need a repeat intervention, as they are still asymptomatic. TLR continues to be one of the strongest clinical endpoint for understanding restenosis because it relates to patient symptoms.

Drug-eluting stents

A drug-eluting stent (DES) consists of three major components (Figure 4.8):

- The metallic stent and delivery balloon catheter.
- The primer layer which maintains polymer integrity.
- The polymer-drug carrier layer, which acts as both a drug reservoir and to prolong drug release. The released anti-proliferative drug inhibits new tissue growth within the sub-intima (neo-intimal hyperplasia), preventing in-stent restenosis (Figure 4.9).

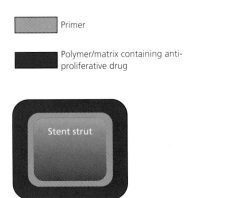

Figure 4.8 Cross-section of a drug-eluting stent strut showing layering of primer used to maintain polymer integrity and polymer matrix, which acts as a reservoir for the anti-proliferative drug and allows its controlled release.

Compared to BMS, DES significantly reduces rates of restenosis (2–4%) and has therefore rapidly become the standard of care for the treatment of coronary artery disease. The very low angiographic and clinical restenosis rates associated with DES has translated to far fewer episodes of recurrent angina and ischaemia requiring repeat PCI or CABG. This is important as in-stent restenosis is not always a benign event. In one study, 9.5% of patients with in-stent restenosis presented with acute myocardial infarction and 26.4% with unstable angina. Furthermore, the PCI or CABG procedure required to treat symptomatic restenosis may also result in myocardial infarction and death.

The first generation stents – Cypher and Taxus – are coated respectively with sirolimus (an immunosuppressant used to prevent renal rejection, which inhibits smooth muscle proliferation and reduces intimal thickening after vascular injury) and paclitaxel (the active component of the anti-cancer drug taxol). More recent second-generation stents, constructed from thinner stainless steel alloy struts and containing more biocompatible polymers, are coated with everolimus (Xience V, Promus, Promus Element), biolimus (Biomatrix) and zotarolimus (Endeavor, Resolute).

The ability of DESs to inhibit neointimal hyperplasia has led to a new measure – *late lumen loss* – which is a precise angiographic representation of this process and a good measure of DES effectiveness. Calculation of late loss, measured in millimetres, is calculated by subtracting the follow-up *minimum lumen diameter* (MLD) from the post-procedure MLD.

Late stent thrombosis

Thrombus formation within a deployed stent in the acute stage (up to 30 days) is rare but may be a catastrophic complication with a mortality of up to 40%. It can happen in patients receiving both bare metal and DESs. It may be associated with

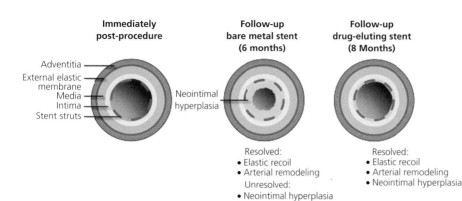

Figure 4.9 Differing mechanism between bare metal and drug-eluting stents in prevention of stent restenosis.

a sub-optimal angiographic result, high-risk lesion characteristics (such as bifurcation, small vessels or thrombotic lesions), diabetes, malignancy, renal failure, antiplatelet non-responders or their early cessation (currently, aspirin and clopidogrel or prasugrel).

In 2006, first-generation DESs were linked to a slightly higher rate of *late stent thrombosis* (>30 days to 1 year) compared to BMS. It attracted much media coverage, controversy and concern among clinicians and patients. However, subsequent data from numerous trials and registries have shown that whilst there probably was a greater risk of late stent thrombosis with first-generation DES, this was not associated with significant increases in death or myocardial infarction when compared to BMS. They were durably associated with reductions in restenosis related end points.

Late stent thrombosis may be the result of a number of risk factors (Figure 4.10). These may include a combination of polymer coating integrity setbacks on the stent metal surface, delayed arterial healing characterised by persistent fibrin deposition, incomplete re-endothelialisation and local hypersensitivity reaction related to the anti-proliferative drug and polymer coating (Figure 4.11). For these reasons, additional improvements have been made to second-generation stents such as a more biocompatible polymer (phosphorylcholine polymer with zotarolimus in the Endeavor stent and a stable fluoropolymer with everolimus in the Xience V, Promus, Promus Element stents). Other improvements include

a biodegradable polymer with abluminal coating (Biomatrix), polymer-free drug delivery, a prohealing approach and the fully biodegradable stent. Recent data shows that second generation drug eluting stents are at least as effective as first generation DES, with no significant increase in late (or very late) stent thrombosis rate.

Perioperative care of patients with stents

Non-cardiac surgery in patients who have undergone recent PCI are at increased risk of stent thrombosis, especially if dual antiplatelet therapy is discontinued. Most stent thromboses occur during or soon after the surgical procedure and in view of the associated high morbidity and death, strategies to minimise the risk are very important.

Where possible, PCI should be avoided before non-cardiac surgery. If PCI is necessary, the type of stent (BMS or DES) should be carefully considered as the former requires dual antiplatelet therapy for 1 month only followed by aspirin alone, whereas the latter requires dual antiplatelet therapy for 12 months, followed by aspirin alone. If PCI has been performed, surgery should be delayed until clopidogrel/prasugrel can be safely discontinued. Unless the risk of bleeding during surgery is prohibitively high, aspirin should be continued where possible.

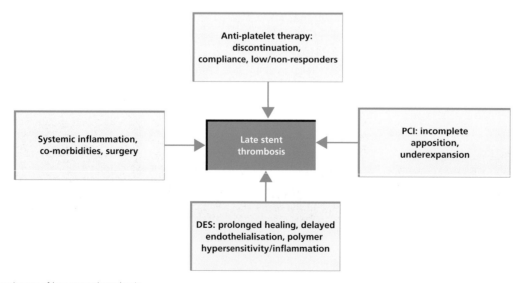

Figure 4.10 Determinants of late stent thrombosis.

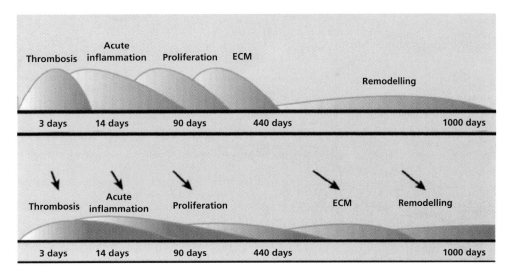

Figure 4.11 The healing course associated with stent injury following bare metal (top) and first-generation drug-eluting stents (bottom). Five distinct stages are present that may last beyond 18 months. Although drug-eluting stents successfully suppress smooth muscle cell proliferation and extracellular matrix, they are associated with a delay in both endothelialisation and inflammatory response beyond 90 days. More modern stents have better biocompatibility and cause less inflammation minimising the time course of thrombus and inflammatory stages, whilst continuing to suppress neointimal proliferation and allow a more complete and functional endothelium (ECM, extracellular matrix; remodelling, compensatory intimal shrinkage).

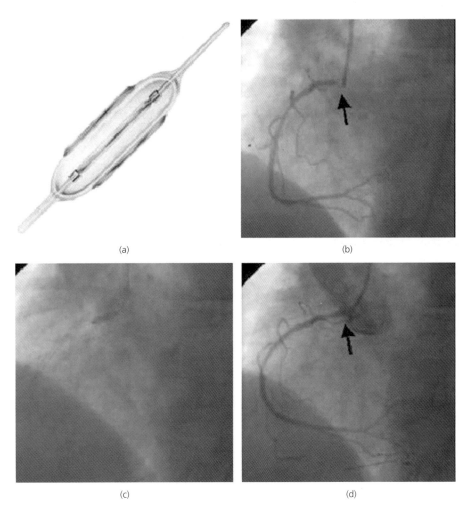

Figure 4.12 The cutting balloon catheter. The longitudinal cutting blades are exposed only during balloon inflation (a). In this case (b), a severe ostial in-stent restenosis in the right coronary artery (arrow) was dilated with a short cutting balloon (c), and a good angiographic result was obtained (arrow, (d)).

In-stent restenosis

Although DESs have markedly reduced the incidence of in-stent restenosis, there remains a small percentage of patients in whom this occurs. Use of repeat percutaneous balloon angioplasty (with or without another stent) to re-dilate in-stent restenosis is feasible but results in a high recurrence of further restenosis (60%). Various other methods, such as removing restenotic tissue by means of atherectomy or a laser device or re-dilating with a cutting balloon (Figure 4.12), have been evaluated, but the results have been disappointing. Another method is brachytherapy, which uses a special intracoronary catheter to deliver a source of β or γ radiation. It significantly reduces further in-stent restenosis, but it has limitations, including late thrombosis and new restenosis at the edges of the radiation-treated segments, giving rise to a 'candy wrapper' appearance (Figure 4.13). Brachytherapy has now been superseded by DESs when a new DES stent is deployed inside the previous stent (Figure 4.14).

Occupation and driving

Doctors may be asked to advise on whether a patient is 'fit for work' or 'recovered from an event' after PCI. 'Fitness' depends on clinical factors (level of symptoms, extent and severity of coronary

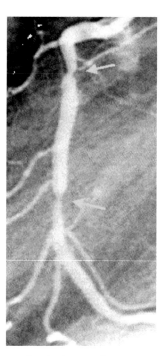

Figure 4.13 Angiogram showing late 'candy wrapper' edge effect (arrows) because of new restenosis at the edges of a segment treated by brachytherapy.

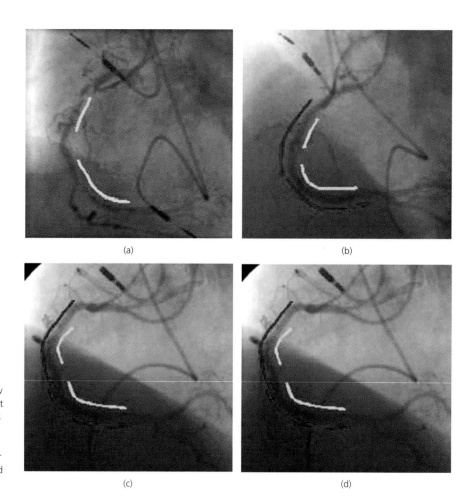

(a)

(b)

(c)

(d)

Figure 4.14 (a) Four months after two stents (yellow lines) were deployed in the proximal and middle right coronary artery, severe diffuse in-stent restenosis has occurred with recurrent angina. (b) Two sirolimus-coated Cypher stents (red lines) were deployed within the original stents. ((c) and (d)) After 6 months, there was no recurrence of restenosis, and the 51-year old patient remained asymptomatic.

disease, left ventricular function, stress test result) and the nature of the occupation, as well as statutory and non-statutory fitness requirements. Advisory medical standards are in place for certain occupations, such as in the armed forces and police, railwaymen and professional divers. Statutory requirements cover the road, marine and aviation industries and some recreational pursuits such as driving and flying.

Patients often ask when they may resume driving after PCI. In Britain, the Driver and Vehicle Licensing Agency recommends that group 1 (private motor car) licence holders should stop driving when anginal symptoms occur at rest or at the wheel. After PCI, they should not drive for a week. Drivers holding a group 2 licence (lorries or buses) will be disqualified from driving once the diagnosis of angina has been made, and for at least 6 weeks after PCI. Relicensing may be permitted provided the exercise test requirement (satisfactory completion of 9 minutes of the Bruce protocol while not taking β-blockers) can be met and there is no other disqualifying condition.

Further reading

Almond DG. Coronary stenting I: intracoronary stents-form, function future. In: Grech ED, Ramsdale DR, eds. *Practical Interventional Cardiology*. 2nd ed. London: Martin Dunitz, 2002:63–76.

Chen MS, John JM, Chew DP, Lee DS, Ellis SG, Bhatt DL. Bare metal stent restenosis is not a benign clinical entity. *Am Heart J* 2006;**151**(**6**):1260–64.

Kimmel SE, Berlin JA, Laskey WK. The relationship between coronary angioplasty procedure volume and major complications. *JAMA* 1995;**274**: 1137–42.

Morice MC, Serruys PW, Sousa JE *et al.* A randomized comparison of a sirolimus-eluting stent with a standard stent for coronary revascularization. *N Engl J Med* 2002;**346**:1773–80.

Settler C, Wandell S, Alleman S *et al.* Outcomes associated with drug-eluting and bare metal stents: a collaborative network meta-analysis. *Lancet* 2007; **370**:937–48.

Smith SC Jr, Dove JT, Jacobs AK *et al.* ACC/AHA guidelines of percutaneous coronary interventions (revision of the 1993 PTCA guidelines) – executive summary. A report of the American College of Cardiology/American Heart Association Task Force on Practice Guidelines (committee to revise the 1993 guidelines for percutaneous transluminal coronary angioplasty). *J Am Coll Cardiol* 2001;**37**:2215–39.

Waksman R. Management of restenosis through radiation therapy. In: Grech ED, Ramsdale DR, eds. *Practical Interventional Cardiology*. 2nd ed. London: Martin Dunitz, 2002:295–305.

CHAPTER 5

Chronic Stable Angina: Treatment Options

Laurence O'Toole and Ever D. Grech

South Yorkshire Cardiothoracic Centre, Northern General Hospital, Sheffield, UK

OVERVIEW

- Anti-anginal drugs, percutaneous coronary intervention (PCI) and coronary artery bypass graft (CABG) surgery are the three principal treatment options for treating chronic stable angina. All aim to reduce myocardial ischaemia and anginal symptoms

- In some subsets of patients, CABG may provide an additional prognostic benefit compared with medical therapy

- Factors influencing the choice of PCI or CABG are varied and complex

- In general, PCI is indicated for single- and two-vessel coronary disease, whereas CABG may be the treatment of choice in more extensive two- and three-vessel disease

- Drug-eluting stents allow a greater number of patients to be treated with PCI instead of CABG

- Alternative therapies attempt to provide symptom improvement in those patients who are unresponsive to both maximal medical therapy and revascularisation techniques

---

In patients with chronic stable angina, factors influencing the choice of coronary revascularisation therapy (percutaneous coronary intervention (PCI) or coronary artery bypass graft (CABG) surgery) are varied and complex. The severity of symptoms, lifestyle, extent of objective ischaemia and underlying risks must be weighed against the benefits of revascularisation and the patient's preference, as well as local availability and expertise. Evidence from randomised trials and large revascularisation registers can guide these decisions, but the past decade has seen rapid changes in medical treatment, bypass surgery and percutaneous intervention. Therefore, thought must be given to whether older data still apply to contemporary practice.

Patients with chronic stable angina have an average annual mortality of 1–3%, only twice that of age-matched controls, and this relatively benign prognosis is an important consideration when determining the merits of revascularisation treatment. Certain patients, however, are at much higher risk (Table 5.1). Predictors include poor exercise capacity with easily inducible ischaemia or a poor haemodynamic response to exercise, angina of recent onset,

Table 5.1 Major factors influencing risks and benefits of coronary revascularisation.

- Advanced age
- Female
- Severe angina
- Smoking
- Diabetes
- Obesity
- Hypertension
- Multiple coronary vessels affected
- Coexisting valve disease
- Impaired left ventricular function
- Impaired renal function
- Cerebrovascular or peripheral vascular disease
- Recent acute coronary syndrome
- Chronic obstructive pulmonary disease

---

previous myocardial infarction, impaired left ventricular function and the number of coronary vessels with significant stenoses, especially when disease affects the left main stem or proximal left anterior descending artery. Although the potential benefits of revascularisation must be weighed against adverse factors, those most at risk may have the most to gain.

Treatment strategies

Medical treatment

Lifestyle modification and drug therapy are important therapeutic interventions in chronic stable angina. Smoking cessation, regular exercise and weight and blood pressure control are mandatory advice for all angina patients and impact significantly on future risk.

Anti-ischaemic drugs improve symptoms and quality of life, but have not been shown to reduce mortality or myocardial infarction. β-blockers may improve survival in hypertension, in heart failure and after myocardial infarction, and so are considered by many to be first-line treatment. Nicorandil has been shown to reduce ischaemic events and the need for hospital admission. Newer agents, such as ivabradine and ranolazine, may also be considered in certain subsets of patients.

Many trials comparing medical treatment with revascularisation predated the widespread use of antiplatelet and cholesterol-lowering drugs. These drugs reduce risk, both in patients treated with

ABC of Interventional Cardiology, 2nd edition.
© Ever D. Grech. Published 2011 Blackwell Publishing Ltd.

drugs only and in those undergoing revascularisation, and so may have altered the risk–benefit ratio for a particular revascularisation strategy in some patients. The more recent COURAGE study has emphasised the importance of both anti-ischaemic and risk-factor-modifying drugs – whether revascularisation was performed or not.

Coronary artery bypass graft (CABG) surgery

Coronary artery bypass graft (CABG) surgery involves the placement of grafts to bypass stenosed native coronary arteries, while maintaining cerebral and peripheral circulation by cardiopulmonary bypass (Figure 5.1). The grafts are usually saphenous veins or arteries (principally the left internal mammary artery and also the right internal mammary and radial artery conduits).

Operative mortality is generally 1–2% but may be much higher in certain subsets of patients. Scoring systems can predict operative mortality based on clinical, investigational and operative factors (Table 5.2). Important developments that have occurred since trials of bypass surgery versus medical treatment were conducted include increased use of arterial grafts, which have much greater longevity than venous grafts, surgery without extracorporeal circulation ('off pump' bypass) and minimal access surgery.

Percutaneous coronary intervention (PCI)

The main advantages of percutaneous intervention over bypass surgery are the avoidance of the risks of general anaesthesia, uncomfortable sternotomy and saphenous wounds, complications

Table 5.2 Risk score for assessing probable mortality from bypass surgery in patients with chronic stable angina.

Risk factor	Weighted score
Age >60	Score 1 for every 5 years over
Female sex	1
Chronic obstructive pulmonary disease	1
Extracardiac arteriopathy	2
Neurological dysfunction	2
Previous cardiac surgery	3
Serum creatinine >200 µmol/l	2
Reduced left ventricular ejection fraction	1 for 30–50% 3 for <30%
Myocardial infarction in past 90 days	2
Pulmonary artery systolic pressure >60 mm Hg	2
Major cardiac procedure as well as bypass surgery	2
Emergency operation	2

Total score ≤2 predicts <1% operative mortality. Total score of 3–5 predicts 3% operative mortality. Total score ≥6 predicts >10% operative mortality. A more detailed assessment with logistic analysis is available at www.euroscore.org and is recommended for assessing high-risk patients.

of major surgery (infections and pulmonary emboli) and stroke. Only an overnight hospital stay is necessary (and some may be performed as day cases), and the procedure can be easily repeated. The mortality is very low (0.2%) and the most serious late complication is restenosis. The advent of drug-eluting stents has significantly reduced the latter from around 20% to less than 5%.

Patient suitability is primarily determined by technical factors. A focal stenosis on a straight artery without proximal vessel tortuousness or involvement of major side branches is ideal for percutaneous intervention. Long, heavily calcified stenoses in tortuous vessels or at bifurcations and chronic total occlusions are less suitable. This must be borne in mind when interpreting data from trials of percutaneous intervention and bypass surgery, as only a minority of patients were suitable for both procedures. Nowadays, more and more patients undergo percutaneous intervention, and referral rates for bypass surgery continue to fall.

PCI also lends itself to patients who have already undergone bypass surgery. It can be carried out in diseased vein grafts (Figure 5.2) and other conduits as well as in diseased, previously grafted native coronary arteries when the graft has failed.

Comparative studies of revascularisation strategies

Coronary artery bypass surgery versus medical treatment

In a meta-analysis of seven trials comparing bypass surgery with medical treatment, surgery conferred a survival advantage in patients with severe left main stem coronary disease, three-vessel disease or two-vessel disease with severely affected proximal left anterior descending artery. The survival gain was more pronounced in patients with left ventricular dysfunction or a strongly positive exercise test (Table 5.3). However, only 10% of trial patients received an internal mammary artery graft, only 25% received antiplatelet drugs and the benefit of lipid-lowering drugs on long-term graft patency was not appreciated when these studies were carried out. Furthermore, 40% of the medically

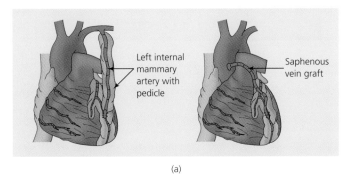

(a)

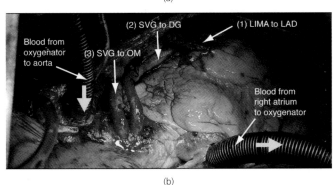

(b)

Figure 5.1 (a) Diagrams of saphenous vein and left internal mammary artery grafts for coronary artery bypass surgery. (b) Three completed grafts – (1) left internal mammary artery (LIMA) to left anterior descending artery (LAD), and saphenous vein grafts (SVG) to (2) diagonal artery (DG) and (3) obtuse marginal artery (OM).

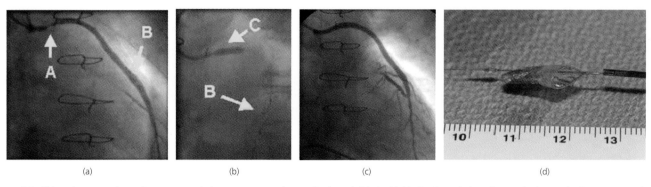

(a)　　　　　　　(b)　　　　　　　(c)　　　　　　　(d)

Figure 5.2 Old saphenous vein grafts may contain large amounts of necrotic clotted debris, friable laminated thrombus and ulcerated atheromatous plaque and are unattractive for percutaneous intervention because of the high risk of distal embolisation. However, distal embolisation protection devices such as the FilterWire (d) reduce this risk by trapping any material released. Such a device (arrow B) in (a) is positioned in the distal segment of a subtotally occluded saphenous vein graft of the left anterior descending artery (arrow A) before it is dilated and stented (arrow C) in (b) to restore blood flow (c).

Table 5.3 Subgroup analysis of mortality benefit from coronary artery bypass surgery compared with medical treatment at 10 years after randomisation for patients with chronic stable angina.

Subgroup	Mean (1.96 SE) increased survival time (months)	p value of difference
Vessel disease:		
1 or 2 vessels	1.8 (3.0)	0.25
3 vessels	5.7 (3.6)	0.001
Left main stem	19.3 (13.7)	0.005
Left ventricular function:		
Normal	2.3 (2.4)	0.06
Abnormal	10.6 (6.1)	<0.001
Exercise test:		
Normal	3.3 (4.4)	0.14
Abnormal	5.1 (3.3)	0.002
Severity of angina:		
CCS class 0, I, II	3.3 (2.7)	0.02
CCS class III, IV	7.3 (4.8)	0.002

CCS, Canadian Cardiovascular Society; SE, standard error.

treated patients underwent bypass surgery during 10 years of follow-up. Thus, these data may underestimate the benefits of surgery compared with medical treatment alone.

In lower risk patients, bypass surgery is indicated only for symptom relief and to improve the quality of life when medical treatment has failed. Surgery does this effectively, with 95% of patients gaining immediate relief from angina and 75% remaining free from angina after 5 years. Unfortunately, venous grafts degenerate over time and have a median life span of only 7–10 years (Figure 5.3). After 15 years, only 15% of patients are free from recurrent angina or death or myocardial infarction. However, the increased use of internal mammary artery grafts, which have excellent long-term patency (85% at 10 years), has increased post-operative survival and reduced long-term symptoms.

Percutaneous coronary intervention versus medical treatment

Most percutaneous procedures are undertaken to treat single-vessel or two-vessel disease, but few randomised controlled studies have compared percutaneous intervention with medical treatment. These showed that patients undergoing the percutaneous

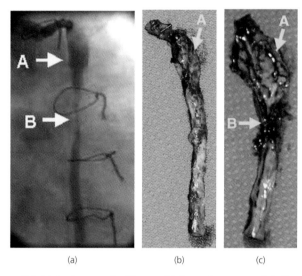

(a)　　　　　(b)　　　　　(c)

Figure 5.3 (a) Angiogram of a 10-year-old diseased venous graft to the obtuse marginal artery showing proximal aneurysmal dilatation (arrow A) and severe stenosis in middle segment (arrow B). (b) Removal of this graft after repeat bypass surgery shows its gross appearance and (c) graft longitudinally opened, with atherosclerosis in a thin-walled aneurysm and a small residual lumen.

procedure derived greater angina relief and took fewer drugs but required more subsequent procedures and had more complications (including non-fatal myocardial infarction), with no mortality difference. Overall, percutaneous coronary intervention does not prevent subsequent death or myocardial infarction in patients with chronic stable angina and well preserved left ventricular function. In contrast to its role in acute coronary syndromes, it should not be considered part of secondary prevention. Therefore, percutaneous intervention is suitable for patients with poor symptom control with drugs and conversely the procedure may not be indicated if symptoms are well controlled.

Percutaneous intervention versus bypass surgery
Single-vessel disease

In a meta-analysis by Pocock *et al.*, percutaneous intervention in patients with single-vessel disease resulted in mortality similar to that found with bypass surgery (3.7% vs 3.1% respectively) but a higher rate of non-fatal myocardial infarction (10.11% vs 6.1%, $p = 0.04$). Angina was well treated in both groups, but persistence of symptoms was slightly higher with percutaneous intervention. Rates of repeat revascularisation were much higher with percutaneous intervention than with bypass surgery.

Lesions within the proximal left anterior descending artery are of particular prognostic importance as this vessel supplies a larger myocardial territory than the left circumflex and right coronary artery combined. Randomised studies comparing percutaneous intervention with conventional or minimally invasive direct coronary artery bypass (MIDCAB) surgery showed no significant mortality difference.

Multivessel disease

Since comparative trials could recruit only those patients who were suitable for either revascularisation strategy, only 3–7% of screened patients were included. These were predominantly 'low-risk' patients with two-vessel disease and preserved left ventricular function – patients in whom bypass surgery has not been shown to improve survival – and therefore it is unlikely that a positive effect in favour of percutaneous intervention would have been detected. The generally benign prognosis of chronic stable angina means that much larger trials would have been required to show significant differences in mortality.

A 2007 meta-analysis of 23 randomised controlled studies comparing PCI with bypass surgery revealed similar short (approximately 96%) and longer term survival rates (approximately 90%) at 5 years and this did not differ significantly between older (>65 years) and younger patients or between those with single- or multivessel disease. Repeat revascularisation rates were higher with PCI (although there was only one small trial using drug-eluting stents). However, the risk of stroke was twice as high with bypass surgery as with PCI (1.2% vs 0.6%).

The nature of percutaneous coronary intervention has changed considerably over the past 10 years, with important developments including the use of drug-eluting stents and improved antiplatelet drugs. The integrated use of these treatments clearly improves outcomes, but almost all of the revascularisation trials predate these developments.

A more recent trial comparing percutaneous intervention and stenting with bypass surgery in multivessel disease confirmed similar rates of death, myocardial infarction and stroke at 1 year, with much lower rates of repeat revascularisation after percutaneous intervention compared with earlier trials. There was also a cost benefit of nearly $3000 (£1875) per patient associated with percutaneous intervention at 12 months. The introduction of drug-eluting stents, which reduce substantially the problem of restenosis, has markedly extended the use of percutaneous intervention in multivessel disease over the last few years, supported by data from large randomised trials such as SYNTAX. This study randomised 1800 patients with *de novo* three-vessel and/or left main coronary artery disease to undergo PCI using taxol-eluting Taxus stents or bypass surgery. At 2 years, the incidence of primary end points of death, stroke, myocardial infarction or repeat revascularisation

was significantly higher for PCI than for bypass surgery, which was mainly driven by higher repeat revascularisation in the PCI arm (17.4% vs 8.6%, $p < 0.001$) as well as a higher rate of myocardial infarction (5.9% vs 3.3%, $p < 0.01$). There was no significant difference in mortality (PCI: 6.2% vs bypass surgery: 4.9%, $p = 0.24$) and stroke rates were significantly higher with bypass surgery (PCI: 1.4% v 2.8% $p < 0.03$). A major contribution of this trial has been the development of the SYNTAX score, which is a useful tool to guide surgeons and cardiologists on revascularisation decisions. The score is based on the presence or absence of specific criteria. These include the number, length and location of lesions, left main stem disease, three-vessel disease, total occlusions, tortuosity, bifurcation or trifurcation, aorto-ostial lesions, thrombus, calcification, diffuse disease and dominance. Details can be obtained from http://www.syntaxscore.com. Analysis of the 2-year outcome data according to baseline SYNTAX score suggests that patients with low (<22) or intermediate (23–32) scores have similar outcomes with PCI or bypass surgery, whereas in those with a high score (≥33) bypass surgery remains the standard of care. The long-term outcome data from the SYNTAX trial are expected to answer many important questions about the relative merits of bypass surgery and PCI in multivessel coronary artery disease and are awaited with interest.

Diabetes

This is an important group of patients as the prevalence of diabetes is increasing and currently stands at around 8% of adults. Cardiovascular complications account for as many as 80% of deaths. Approximately one quarter of all patients referred for revascularisation are diabetic.

Previous studies showed that bypass surgery conferred a survival advantage in symptomatic diabetic patients with multivessel disease. The BARI trial revealed a significant difference in 5-year mortality (21% with percutaneous intervention vs 6% with bypass surgery). Similar trends have been found in other large trials. However, the RAVEL and SIRIUS studies, in which the sirolimus-eluting Cypher stent was compared with the same stent uncoated, showed a remarkable reduction in restenosis rate within the stented segments in diabetic patients (0% vs 42% and 18% vs 51% respectively).

Recent randomised studies comparing PCI using drug-eluting stents with CABG suggest greater equipoise between the two strategies. The SYNTAX trial found similar mortality rates for the two therapies at 2 years in patients with diabetes and low-to-intermediate SYNTAX scores.

The CARDia study was confined to diabetic patients with multivessel disease randomised to PCI or bypass surgery and 510 patients were recruited. Initially, bare metal stents were used and a switch to the sirolimus-eluting Cypher stent was made when these became available. About 69% of patients in the PCI group received a Cypher stent. Although the study was underpowered to meet its primary outcome (a composite of mortality, myocardial infarction and stroke), 1-year results showed similar mortality rates at 3.2% and a statistically significant higher rate of repeat revascularisation in the PCI group (11.8% vs 2.0%) and stoke rate trend favouring

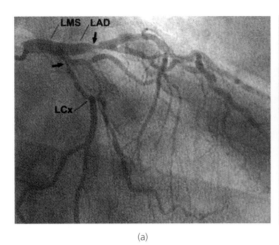
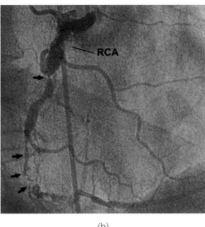

(a)   (b)

Figure 5.4 Coronary angiograms of a 69-year-old man with limiting angina and exertional breathlessness. There was severe proximal disease (arrows) of the left anterior descending (LAD) and left circumflex arteries (LCx) (a) and occlusion of the right coronary artery (RCA) (b). The patient was referred for coronary artery bypass surgery on prognostic and symptomatic grounds.

PCI (0.4% vs 2.8%). Longer term follow-up of these trial data and other ongoing trials will provide further information on optimal strategies for coronary revascularisation in diabetic patients. In particular, the ongoing FREEDOM trial plans to enroll approximately 2000 patients. The primary end point is a composite of all-cause mortality, non-fatal MI and stroke at 5 years.

Other study data

Large registries of outcomes in patients undergoing revascularisation have the advantage of including all patients rather than the highly selected groups included in randomised trials. The registry data seem to agree with those from randomised trials: patients with more extensive disease fare better with bypass surgery (Figure 5.4), whereas percutaneous intervention is preferable in focal coronary artery disease (Figures 5.5 and 5.6).

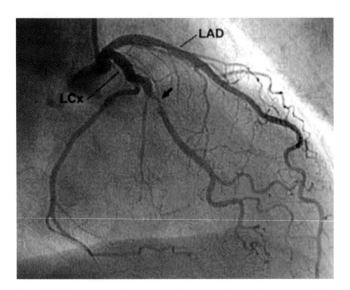

Figure 5.5 Coronary angiogram showing a severe focal stenosis (arrow) in a large oblique marginal branch of the left circumflex artery (LCx), suitable for percutaneous coronary intervention. The left anterior descending artery (LAD) has no significant disease.

An unusual observation is that patients screened and considered suitable for inclusion in a trial fared slightly better if they refused to participate than did those who enrolled. The heterogeneous nature of coronary disease means that certain patient subsets will probably benefit more from one treatment than another. The better outcome in the patients who were suitable but not randomised may indicate that cardiologists and surgeons recognise which patients will benefit more from a particular strategy – subtleties that are lost in the randomisation process of controlled trials.

Left main stem disease

The superiority of bypass surgery over medical treatment for left main stem stenosis has been demonstrated in subgroup analysis of large randomised studies. However, there is little data comparing bypass surgery with percutaneous intervention. Recent results achieved with drug-eluting stents in elective patients have been encouraging. Nevertheless, the recurrence rates remain high in bifurcation lesions and stent thrombosis is still particularly dangerous. Until more data becomes available, percutaneous intervention for unprotected main stem stenosis (when neither the left anterior descending nor the left circumflex arteries is bypassed) is currently reserved for individual cases in which the stenosis is favourable or when bypass surgery would be too high risk. Application of the SYNTAX score may be useful in this setting.

Refractory coronary artery disease

Increasing numbers of patients with coronary artery disease have angina that is unresponsive to both maximal drug treatment and revascularisation techniques. Many will have already undergone multiple percutaneous interventions or bypass surgery procedures, or have diffuse and distal coronary artery disease. In addition to functional limitations, their prognosis may be poor because of impaired ventricular function. Emerging treatments seek to provide alternative methods of symptom improvement but their efficacy remains unclear (Table 5.4).

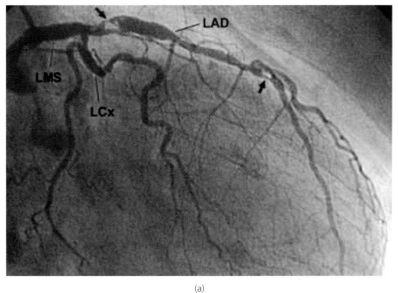
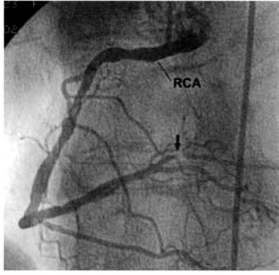

(a)   (b)

Figure 5.6 Coronary angiograms of a 70-year-old woman with limiting angina. (a) There were severe stenoses (arrows) in the proximal and middle left anterior descending artery (LAD) and (b) in the distal right coronary artery (RCA). Because of the focal nature of these lesions, percutaneous coronary intervention was the preferred option.

Table 5.4 Treatment options for refractory angina.

- *Drugs* – analgesics, statins, angiotensin-converting enzyme inhibitors, antiplatelet drugs, amiodarone, ranolazine
- *Neurostimulation* – interruption or modification of afferent nociceptive signals: transcutaneous electric nerve stimulation (TENS), implantable spinal cord stimulation (SCS)
- *Neuroblockade* – left stellate ganglion blockade (LSGB), endoscopic thoracoscopic symathectomy (ETS)
- *Enhanced external counterpulsation* (EECP) – non-invasive pneumatic leg compression, improving coronary perfusion and decreasing left ventricular afterload
- *Laser revascularisation* – small myocardial channels created by laser beams: transmyocardial laser revascularisation (TMLR) and percutaneous transmyocardial laser revascularisation (PTMLR)
- *Therapeutic angiogenesis* – cytokines, vascular endothelial growth factor and fibroblast growth factor injected into ischaemic myocardium, or adenoviral vector for gene transport to promote neovascularisation
- *Intramyocardial bone marrow injection* – the intramyocardial injection of autologous bone marrow cells
- *Percutaneous in situ coronary venous arterialisation (PICVA)* – flow redirection from diseased coronary artery into adjacent coronary vein, causing arterialisation of the vein and retroperfusion into ischaemic myocardium
- *Percutaneous in situ coronary artery bypass (PICAB)* – flow redirection from diseased artery into adjacent coronary vein and then rerouting back into the artery after the lesion
- *Coronary sinus reducer* – an implantable stent designed to narrow the coronary sinus to redistribute blood from non-ischaemic to ischaemic regions of the heart
- *Heart transplantation* – may be considered when all alternative treatments have failed

Further reading

Boden WE, O'Rourke RA, Teo KK, *et al.* Optimal medical therapy with or without PCI for stable coronary disease. *N Engl J Med* 2007;**356**(15):1503–16.

Hlatky MA, Boothroyd B, Bravata DM, *et al.* Coronary artery bypass surgery compared with percutaneous coronary interventions for multivessel disease: a collaborative analysis of individual patient data from ten randomised trials. *Lancet* 2009;**373**:1190–97.

Kim MC, Kini A, Sharma SK. Refractory angina pectoris. Mechanisms and therapeutic options. *J Am Coll Cardiol* 2002;**39**:923–34.

Pocock SJ, Henderson RA, Rickards AF, *et al.* Meta-analysis of randomised trials comparing coronary angioplasty with bypass surgery. *Lancet* 1995;**345**:1184–9.

Raco DL, Yusuf S. Overview of randomised trials of percutaneous coronary intervention: comparison with medical and surgical therapy for chronic coronary artery disease. In: Grech ED, Ramsdale DR, eds. *Practical Interventional Cardiology.* 2nd ed. London: Martin Dunitz, 2002:263–77.

Scottish Intercollegiate Guidelines Network. *Coronary Revascularisation in the Management of Stable Angina Pectoris.* Edinburgh: SIGN, 1998 (SIGN Publication No 32).

Serruys PW, Morice MC, Kappetein AP, *et al.* Percutaneous coronary intervention versus coronary-artery bypass grafting for severe coronary artery disease. *N Engl J Med* 2009;**360**:961–72.

Trikalinos TA, Alsheikh-Ali AA, Tatsioni A, Nallamothu BK, Kent DM. Percutaneous coronary interventions for non-acute coronary artery disease: a quantitative 20-year synopsis and a network meta-analysis. *Lancet* 2009;**373**:911–18.

Yusuf S, Zucker D, Peduzzi P, *et al.* Effect of coronary artery bypass graft surgery on survival: overview of 10-year results from randomised trials by the Coronary Artery Bypass Graft Surgery Trialists Collaboration. *Lancet* 1994;**344**:563–70.

CHAPTER 6

Acute Coronary Syndrome: Unstable Angina and Non-ST Segment Elevation Myocardial Infarction

Ever D. Grech

South Yorkshire Cardiothoracic Centre, Northern General Hospital, Sheffield, UK

OVERVIEW

- Patients with unstable angina or acute non-ST segment elevation myocardial infarction require urgent hospital admission and cardiac monitoring
- All patients should be assessed by a cardiologist on the day of presentation
- Evidence indicates that an 'early invasive' strategy is superior to a 'conservative' strategy in higher risk patients
- The TIMI risk score allows identification of higher risk patients who are likely to benefit from aggressive anti-thrombotic therapy, early coronary angiography and revascularisation
- Aggressive risk factor modification is warranted, especially following hospital discharge
- General practitioners have an important role in monitoring patients' risk factors and secondary prevention measures

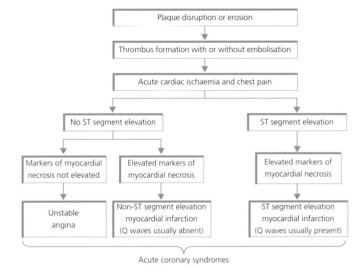

Figure 6.1 Spectrum of acute coronary syndromes according to electrocardiographic and biochemical markers of myocardial necrosis (troponin T or troponin I), in patients presenting with acute cardiac chest pain.

Table 6.1 Three main presentations of unstable angina.

- *Angina at rest* – also prolonged, usually >20 min
- *Angina of new onset* – at least CCS class III in severity
- *Angina increasing* – previously diagnosed angina that has become more frequent, longer in duration or lower in threshold (change in severity by >1 CCS class to at least CCS class III)

CCS, Canadian Cardiovascular Society.

The term *acute coronary syndrome* refers to a range of acute myocardial ischaemic states. It encompasses unstable angina, non-ST segment elevation myocardial infarction (ST segment elevation generally absent) and ST segment elevation infarction (persistent ST segment elevation usually present) – (Figure 6.1). This chapter will focus on the role of percutaneous coronary intervention (PCI) in the management of unstable angina and non-ST segment elevation myocardial infarction; these are collectively referred to as non-ST segment elevation acute coronary syndrome (NSTE-ACS). The next chapter will address the role of percutaneous intervention in acute ST segment elevation myocardial infarction (STEMI).

Although there is no universally accepted definition of unstable angina, it has been described as a clinical syndrome between stable angina and acute myocardial infarction. This broad definition encompasses many patients presenting with varying histories and reflects the complex pathophysiological mechanisms operating at different times and with different outcomes. Three main presentations have been described – angina at rest, new onset angina and increasing angina (Table 6.1).

Pathogenesis

The process central to the initiation of an acute coronary syndrome is disruption of an atheromatous plaque. Fissuring or rupture of these plaques – and consequent exposure of core constituents such as lipid, smooth muscle and foam cells – leads to the local generation of thrombin and deposition of fibrin. This in turn promotes platelet aggregation and adhesion and the formation of intracoronary thrombus (Figure 6.2). Unstable angina and non-ST segment elevation myocardial infarction are generally associated with white, platelet-rich and only partially occlusive thrombus. Microthrombi can detach and embolise downstream, causing

ABC of Interventional Cardiology, 2nd edition.
© Ever D. Grech. Published 2011 Blackwell Publishing Ltd.

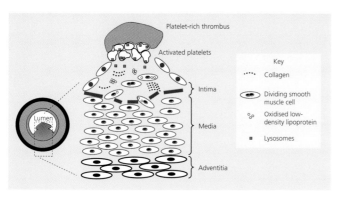

Figure 6.2 Diagram of an unstable plaque with superimposed luminal thrombus.

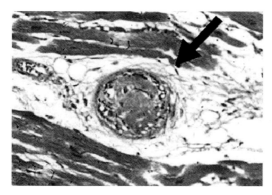

Figure 6.3 Distal embolisation of a platelet-rich thrombus causing occlusion of intramyocardial arteriole (arrow). Such an event may result in microinfarction and elevation of markers of myocardial necrosis.

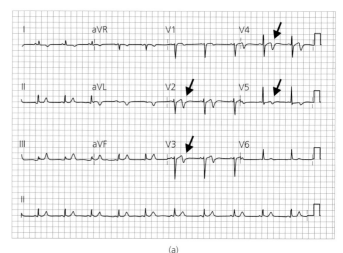

(a)

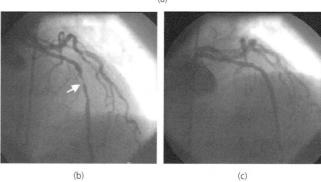

(b)   (c)

Figure 6.4 Electrocardiogram of a 48-year-old woman with unstable angina (a). Note the acute ischaemic changes in leads V1 to V5 (arrows). Coronary angiography revealed a severe mid-left anterior descending coronary artery stenosis (arrow, b), which was successfully stented (c).

myocardial ischaemia and infarction (Figure 6.3). In contrast, ST segment elevation myocardial infarction often has red, fibrin-rich and more stable occlusive thrombus.

Epidemiology

Unstable angina and non-ST segment elevation myocardial infarction account for about 2.5 million hospital admissions worldwide and are a major cause of mortality and morbidity in Western countries. The prognosis is substantially worse than for chronic stable angina. In-hospital death and reinfarction affect 5–10%. Despite optimal treatment with anti-ischaemic and anti-thrombotic drugs, death and recurrent myocardial infarction occur in another 5–10% of patients in the month after an acute episode. Several studies indicate that these patients may have a higher long-term risk of death and myocardial infarction than do patients with ST segment elevation myocardial infarction.

Diagnosis

Unstable angina and non-ST segment elevation myocardial infarction are closely related conditions with clinical presentations that may be indistinguishable. Their distinction depends on whether the ischaemia is severe enough to cause myocardial damage and the release of detectable quantities of markers of myocyte necrosis.

Cardiac troponin I and T are the preferred markers as they are more specific and reliable than creatine kinase or its isoenzyme creatine kinase MB.

An electrocardiogram may be normal or show minor non-specific changes, ST segment depression, T-wave inversion (Figure 6.4), bundle branch block or transient ST segment elevation that resolves spontaneously or after nitrate is given. Physical examination may exclude important differential diagnoses such as pleuritis, pericarditis or pneumothorax, as well as revealing evidence of ventricular failure and haemodynamic instability.

Management

Management has evolved considerably over the past decade. As platelet aggregation and thrombus formation play a key role in acute coronary syndrome, recent advances in treatment (such as the glycoprotein IIb/IIIa inhibitors, low molecular weight heparin, clopidogrel and prasugrel) and the safer and more widespread use of PCI have raised questions about optimal management.

As patients with unstable angina or non-ST segment elevation myocardial infarction represent a heterogeneous group with a wide spectrum of clinical outcomes, tailoring treatment to match risk not only ensures that patients who will benefit the most receive appropriate treatment but also avoids potentially hazardous treatment in those with a good prognosis. Therefore, an accurate diagnosis and estimation of the risk of adverse outcome are prerequisites to selecting the most appropriate treatment. This should begin in the emergency department and continue throughout the hospital admission. Ideally, all patients should be assessed by a cardiologist on the day of presentation.

Medical treatment

In those with probable or confirmed unstable angina or non-ST segment elevation myocardial infarction, medical treatment includes bed rest, oxygen if hypoxic, opiate analgesics to relieve pain, anti-ischaemic and anti-thrombotic drugs. Anti-ischaemic drugs include intravenous, oral or buccal nitroglycerin, β-blockers and calcium antagonists. Anti-thrombotic drugs include aspirin, clopidogrel or prasugrel, intravenous unfractionated heparin or low molecular weight heparin and glycoprotein IIb/IIIa inhibitors. In addition, early initiation of statin therapy has been shown to reduce longer term mortality, unstable angina and the need for revascularisation.

'Conservative' versus 'early invasive' strategies

'Conservative' treatment involves intensive medical management, followed by risk stratification by non-invasive means (usually by stress testing) to identify patients who may need coronary angiography. This approach was based on the results of two randomised trials (TIMI IIIB and VANQWISH), which showed no improvement in outcome when an 'early invasive' strategy was used routinely, compared with a selective approach. These findings generated much controversy and have been superseded by more recent randomised trials, which have taken advantage of the benefits of glycoprotein IIb/IIIa inhibitors and intracoronary stents (Figure 6.5). These studies showed that an early invasive strategy (early angiography followed by PCI or coronary artery bypass surgery) produced significantly better outcomes than non-invasive management (Figures 6.6 and 6.7). TACTICS-TIMI 18 also showed that the benefit of early invasive treatment was greatest in higher risk patients with raised plasma concentrations of troponin T, whereas the outcomes for lower risk patients were similar with early invasive and non-invasive management.

Identifying higher risk patients

Identifying patients at higher risk of death, myocardial infarction and recurrent ischaemia allows aggressive anti-thrombotic

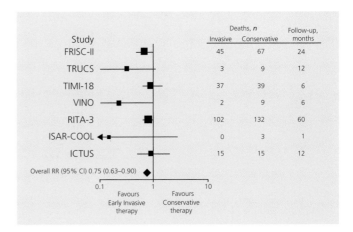

Figure 6.6 Relative risk of all-cause mortality for early invasive compared with conservative strategies at a mean follow-up of 2 years, showing a long-term survival benefit from early invasive therapy (4.9% vs 6.5%, $p = 0.001$).

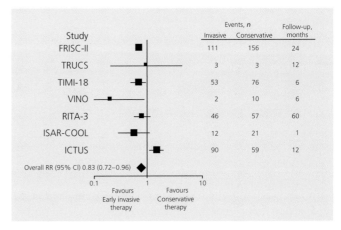

Figure 6.7 Relative risk of recurrent non-fatal myocardial infarction for early invasive compared to conservative strategies at a mean follow-up of 2 years, showing a long-term reduction in myocardial infarction from early invasive therapy (7.6% vs 9.1%, $p = 0.012$).

treatment and early coronary angiography to be targeted to those who will benefit. The initial diagnosis is made on the basis of a patient's history, electrocardiography and the presence of elevated plasma concentrations of biochemical markers of myocardial necrosis. The same information is used to assess the risk of an

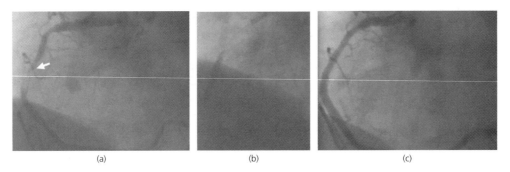

Figure 6.5 Right coronary artery angiogram in patient with non-ST segment elevation myocardial infarction (a), showing hazy appearance of intraluminal thrombus overlying a severe stenosis (arrow). Abciximab was given before direct stenting (b), with good angiographic outcome (c).

Table 6.2 The seven variables for the TIMI risk score.

- Age >65 years
- >3 risk factors for coronary artery disease
- >50% coronary stenosis on angiography
- ST segment change >0.5 mm
- >2 anginal episodes in 24 h before presentation
- Elevated serum concentration of cardiac markers
- Use of aspirin in 7 d before presentation

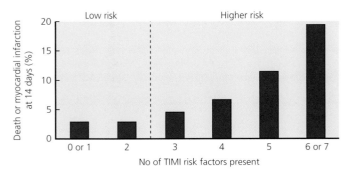

Figure 6.8 Rates of death from all-causes and non-fatal myocardial infarction at 14 days, by TIMI risk score. Note sharp rate increase when score >3.

adverse outcome. It should be emphasised that risk assessment is a continuous process.

The TIMI risk score

Attempts have been made to formulate clinical factors into a user-friendly model. Notably, Antman and colleagues identified seven independent prognostic risk factors for early death and myocardial infarction. Assigning a value of 1 for each risk factor present provides a simple scoring system for estimating risk, the TIMI risk score. It has the advantage of being easy to calculate and has broad applicability in the early assessment of patients (Table 6.2; Figure 6.8).

Applying this score to the results in the TACTICS-TIMI 18 study indicated that patients with a TIMI risk score of ≥3 benefited significantly from an early invasive strategy, whereas those with a score of ≤2 did not. Therefore, those with an initial TIMI score of ≥3 should be considered for early angiography (ideally within 24 hours), with a view to revascularisation by percutaneous intervention or bypass surgery. In addition, any patient with an elevated plasma concentration of troponin marker, ST segment changes or haemodynamic instability should also undergo early angiography (Figure 6.9).

Conclusion

The diagnosis of unstable angina or non-ST segment elevation myocardial infarction demands urgent hospital admission and cardiac monitoring. A clinical history and examination, 12-lead electrocardiography and measurement of troponin concentration are the essential diagnostic tools. Bed rest, oxygen if hypoxic, opiate

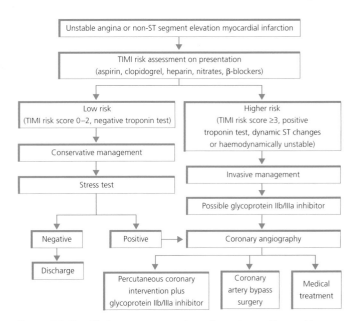

Figure 6.9 Simplified management pathway for patients with unstable angina or non-ST segment elevation myocardial infarction.

analgesics, anti-ischaemic and anti-thrombotic drugs and statins are the mainstay of initial treatment.

Early risk stratification will help identify high-risk patients, who may require early angiography and coronary revascularisation. Those deemed suitable for percutaneous intervention may receive a glycoprotein IIb/IIIa inhibitor (if not already started) as appropriate (Figure 6.7). There are differences in current guidelines on when and who should receive a glycoprotein IIb/IIIa inhibitor (Table 6.3). There seems to be little merit in prolonged stabilisation of patients before angiography, and an early invasive strategy is generally preferable to a conservative one except for patients at low risk of further cardiac events. This approach will shorten hospital

Table 6.3 Guidelines: GP IIb/IIIa in NSTEMI.

European Society of Cardiology
- In intermediate- to high-risk (elevated troponin, ST segment depression or diabetes) eptifibatide or tirofiban for initial early treatment
- In high-risk patients not pretreated with a GP IIb/IIIa inhibitor and proceeding to PCI, abciximab is recommended following angiography
- Use of eptifibatide or tirofiban is less well established
- When anatomy is known and PCI is planned within 24 h with GP IIb/IIIa inhibitor, most secure evidence is for abciximab

American College of Cardiology/American Heart Association
- Initial invasive strategy
- Initiate upstream antiplatelet therapy in addition to aspirin with either clopidogrel or a GP IIb/IIIa inhibitor
- Abciximab only if no appreciable delay to angiography and PCI likely, otherwise eptifibatide or tirofiban

Conservative Strategy
- If recurrent symptoms or ischaemia, heart failure or serious arrhythmia, either a GP IIb/IIIa inhibitor (eptifibatide/tirofiban) or clopidogrel should be added to aspirin and anticoagulant before angiography.

GP IIb/IIIa, Glycoprotein IIb/IIIa; NSTEMI, non-ST segment elevation myocardial infarction; PCI, percutaneous coronary intervention.

stays, improve acute and long-term outcomes and reduce the need for subsequent intervention. Following percutaneous intervention, clopidogrel or prasugrel (especially after stenting) is generally continued for 12 months, apart from life-long aspirin.

In the longer term, aggressive modification of risk factors is warranted. Smoking should be strongly discouraged, and statins should be used to lower blood lipid levels. β-blockers, angiotensin-converting enzyme inhibitors and anti-hypertensive drugs should also be considered. If present, diabetes should be optimally managed. Anti-ischaemic drugs may be stopped when ischaemia provocation tests are negative.

Further reading

Anderson JL, Adams CD, Antman EM *et al*. ACC/AHA 2007 Guidelines for the management of patients with unstable angina/non–ST-elevation myocardial infarction: A report of the American College of Cardiology/ American Heart Association Task Force on practice guidelines. *J Am Coll Cardiol* 2007;**50**:e1–e157.

Antman EM, Cohen M, Bernink PJ *et al*. The TIMI risk score for unstable angina/non-ST elevation MI: a method for prognostication and therapeutic decision making. *JAMA* 2000;**284**:835–42.

Bassand JP, Hamm CW, Ardissino D *et al*. The Task Force for the Diagnosis and Treatment of Non-ST-Segment Elevation Acute Coronary Syndromes of the European Society of Cardiology. Guidelines for the diagnosis and treatment of non-ST-segment elevation acute coronary syndromes. *Eur Heart J* 2007;**28**:1598–660.

Bavry AA, Kumbhani DJ, Rassi AN, Bhatt DL, Askari AT. Benefit of early invasive therapy in acute coronary syndromes: a meta-analysis of contemporary randomized clinical trails. *J Am Coll Cardiol* 2006;**48**: 1319–25.

Ramsdale DR, Grech ED. Percutaneous coronary intervention unstable angina and non-Q-wave myocardial infarction. In: Grech ED, Ramsdale DR, eds. *Practical Interventional Cardiology*. 2nd ed. London: Martin Dunitz, 2002:165–87.

CHAPTER 7

Acute Coronary Syndrome: ST Segment Elevation Myocardial Infarction

Ever D. Grech

South Yorkshire Cardiothoracic Centre, Northern General Hospital, Sheffield, UK

OVERVIEW

- The two main methods of reopening an occluded infarct-related artery are either a thrombolytic agent or primary percutaneous coronary intervention (PCI)

- In some patients, PCI may also be performed after thrombolytic therapy

- Although primary PCI is a superior mode of recanalisation compared to thrombolytic therapy, it can only be performed when adequate facilities and experienced staff are available

- Drug-eluting stents may offer significant additional benefits in reducing recurrent ischaemia and restenosis

- Anti-thrombotic agents given before, during and after primary PCI play an important role in successful short- and long-term outcomes

- Secondary prevention is essential following acute ST elevation myocardial infarction

---

Acute ST segment elevation myocardial infarction usually occurs when thrombus forms on a ruptured atheromatous plaque and occludes an epicardial coronary artery (Figure 7.1). Patient survival depends on several factors, the most important being restoration of brisk antegrade coronary flow, the time taken to achieve this and the sustained patency of the affected artery. The benefits of reperfusion therapy is largely confined to the first 12 hours after symptom onset.

Recanalisation

There are two main methods of reopening an occluded artery: administering a thrombolytic agent or primary percutaneous coronary intervention (*primary PCI*) – which often includes stent deployment (Figure 7.2).

Although thrombolysis is the commonest form of treatment for acute ST segment elevation myocardial infarction, it has important limitations: a rate of recanalisation (restoring normal flow) at 90 minutes of only 55% with streptokinase or 60% with accelerated alteplase; a 5–15% risk of early or late reocclusion leading to acute

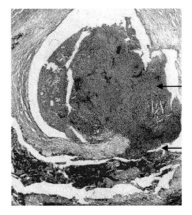

Figure 7.1 Histological appearance of a ruptured atheromatous plaque (bottom arrow) and occlusive thrombus (top arrow) resulting in acute myocardial infarction.

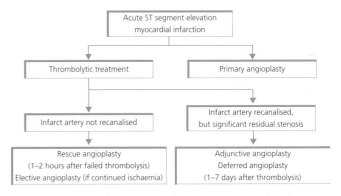

Figure 7.2 Methods of recanalisation for acute ST segment elevation myocardial infarction.

myocardial infarction, worsening ventricular function or death; a 1–2% risk of intracranial haemorrhage with 40% mortality and 15–20% of patients with a contraindication to thrombolysis.

Primary PCI mechanically disrupts the occlusive thrombus and compresses the underlying stenosis, rapidly restoring blood flow. It offers a superior alternative to thrombolysis in the immediate treatment of ST segment elevation myocardial infarction. This differs from sequential angioplasty, when angioplasty is performed after thrombolysis. After early trials of thrombolytic drugs, there was much interest in *facilitated* PCI (angioplasty used as a supplement

---

Table 7.1 Comparison of methods of recanalisation.

	Thrombolysis	Rescue angioplasty	Primary angioplasty
Time from admission to recanalisation	1–3 h after start of thrombolysis	Time to start of thrombolysis plus 2 h	20–60 min
Recanalisation with brisk antegrade flow	55–60%	85%	95%
Systemic fibrinolysis	+++	+++	–
Staff and catheter laboratory 'burden'	–	+	+++
Cost of procedure	+	+++	+++

Table 7.2 Pros and cons of primary PCI compared with thrombolysis.

Advantages
- High patency rates (>90%) with brisk, antegrade flow
- Lower mortality
- Better residual left ventricular function
- More rapid electrocardiographic normalisation
- Less recurrent ischaemia (angina, reinfarction, exercise-induced ischaemia)
- No systemic fibrinolysis, therefore bleeding problems reduced
- Improved risk stratification by angiography with identification of patients suitable for coronary artery bypass surgery or PCI at a later date

Disadvantages
- Higher procedural cost than streptokinase or alteplase (although long-term costs lower)
- Can be performed only when cardiac catheterisation facilities and experienced staff are available
- Recanalisation more rapid than thrombolysis only if 24-h on-call team is available with rapid patient transfer to cath lab
- Risks and complications of cardiac catheterisation and percutaneous intervention
- Reperfusion arrhythmias more common because of more rapid recanalisation

to thrombolysis) as this was expected to reduce recurrent ischaemia and reinfarction. Initial studies (ECSG, TIMI IIB, TAMI), however, not only failed to show any advantage but also found higher rates of major haemorrhage and emergency bypass surgery. In contrast, newer studies have shown conflicting results. On the one hand, two studies (ASSENT-4 and FINESSE) showed that PCI was not beneficial, whereas other studies (CARESS-in-AMI, CAPITAL-AMI and TRANSFER-AMI) showed that it was. The longer delays between symptom onset and thrombolytic therapy may have been a contributory factor. In contrast, *rescue* (also known as salvage) PCI, which is performed if thrombolysis fails to restore patency after 1–2 hours, may confer some benefit (Table 7.1).

Pros and cons of primary PCI

See Table 7.2.

Advantages

Large randomised studies have shown that thrombolysis significantly reduces mortality compared with placebo, and this effect is maintained in the long term. Primary PCI confers additional short- and long-term benefits (Figure 7.3) by way of substantial reductions in rates of death, cerebrovascular events, reinfarction and recurrent ischaemia.

The information provided by immediate coronary angiography is valuable in determining subsequent management. Patients with severe three-vessel disease, severe left main coronary artery stenosis (Figure 7.4) or occluded vessels unsuitable for angioplasty can be referred for urgent bypass surgery. Conversely, patients whose arteries are found to have spontaneously recanalised or who have an insignificant infarct-related artery may be selected for medical treatment, and thus avoid unnecessary thrombolytic treatment. Coronary angiography may also assist in the diagnosis of acute pericarditis, coronary artery spasm and type-A aortic dissection, which may all present with ST segment elevation, and where thrombolytic therapy may be both unnecessary and harmful.

Disadvantages

The morbidity and mortality associated with primary angioplasty is operator dependent, varying with the skill and experience of the interventionist, and it should be considered only for patients

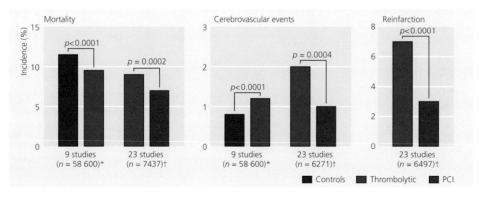

Figure 7.3 Short-term effects of treatment with placebo, thrombolytic drugs or primary PCI on mortality, incidence of cerebrovascular events and incidence of non-fatal reinfarction after acute ST segment elevation myocardial infarction in randomised studies. Of the 1% incidence of cerebrovascular events in patients undergoing primary PCI, only 0.05% was haemorrhagic. In contrast, patients receiving thrombolytic drugs had a 1% incidence of haemorrhagic cerebrovascular events ($p < 0.0001$) and an overall 2% incidence of cerebrovascular events ($p = 0.0004$). *FTT Collaborative Group. *Lancet* 1994;**343**:311–22. †Keeley *et al.* *Lancet* 2003;**361**:13–20.

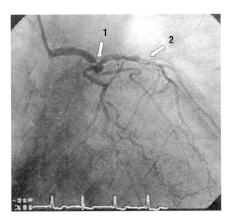

Figure 7.4 Severe distal left main stem stenosis (arrow 1) and partial occlusion of mid-left anterior descending artery due to thrombus (arrow 2). In view of the severity of the lesion, PCI was contraindicated. An intra-aortic balloon pump was used to augment blood pressure and coronary flow before successful bypass surgery.

presenting early (<12 hours after the onset of acute myocardial infarction). Procedural complications are more common than with elective angioplasty for chronic angina, and, even though it is usual to deal only with the occluded vessel, procedures may be prolonged. The presence of a large amount of luminal thrombus is an additional challenge as this may fragment after balloon dilatation or stenting, resulting in distal embolisation which may cause slow- or no-reflow. Ventricular arrhythmias are not unusual on recanalisation, but these generally occur while the patient is still in the catheterisation laboratory and can be promptly treated by intravenous drugs or electrical cardioversion. Right coronary artery procedures are often associated with sinus arrest, atrioventricular block, idioventricular rhythm and severe hypotension. Up to 5% of patients initially referred for primary angioplasty require urgent coronary artery bypass surgery, so surgical backup is essential if risks are to be minimised.

There are logistical hurdles in delivering a full 24-hour service. Primary PCI can be performed only when adequate facilities and experienced staff are available. The time from admission to recanalisation (referred to as the *door to balloon time – D2B*) should be less than 90 minutes, although this can be difficult to achieve as patient transfer times, poor management strategies or other factors can lead to long delays. However, recent evidence suggests that, even with longer delays, primary PCI may still be superior to thrombolysis.

A catheterisation laboratory requires large initial capital expenditure and has substantial running costs. However, in an existing, fully supported laboratory operating at high volume, primary PCI is at least as cost-effective as thrombolysis.

Primary PCI and coronary stents

Although early randomised studies of primary PCI showed its clinical effectiveness, outcomes were marred by high rates of recurrent ischaemia (10–15% of patients) and early reinfarction of the affected artery (up to 5%). Consequently, haemodynamic and arrhythmic complications arose, with the need for repeat catheterisation and revascularisation, prolonged hospital stay and increased costs. Furthermore, restenosis rates in the first 6 months remained disappointingly high (25–45%), and a fifth of patients required revascularisation.

Although stenting the lesion seemed an attractive answer, it was initially thought that deploying a stent in the presence of thrombus over a ruptured plaque would provoke further thrombosis. In fact, one study (Stent-PAMI) showed that stenting was associated with a small (but significant) decrease in normal coronary flow and a trend towards increased 6- and 12-month mortality. This led to the use of adjunctive glycoprotein IIb/IIIa inhibitors as a solution. Further improvements in stent deployment and advances in adjunctive pharmacotherapy have led to greater technical success. Recent studies comparing primary stenting with balloon angioplasty alone have shown that stented patients have significantly less recurrent ischaemia, reinfarction and subsequent need for further angioplasty. Economic analysis has shown that, as expected, the initial costs were higher but were offset by lower follow-up costs after a year.

Since the arrival of drug-eluting stents, there has been some debate about their role in the setting of primary PCI. A systematic review and meta-analysis by Brar *et al.* comparing drug-eluting stents with bare metal stents showed that the former were superior to bare metal stents in preventing recurrent ischaemia due to a reduction in restenosis.

Glycoprotein IIb/IIIa inhibitors and other antiplatelet agents

The potential benefits of intravenous glycoprotein IIb/IIIa inhibitors combined with stenting have been evaluated. The first study (CADILLAC) showed that abciximab significantly reduced early recurrent ischaemia and reocclusion due to thrombus formation. There was no additional effect on restenosis or late outcomes compared with stenting alone. The slightly reduced rate of normal coronary flow that had been seen in other studies was again confirmed, but did not translate into a significant effect on mortality. Another study (ADMIRAL) examined the potential benefit of abciximab when given before (rather than during) primary stenting. Both at 30 days' and 6 months' follow-up, abciximab significantly reduced the composite rate of reinfarction, the need for further revascularisation and mortality. In addition, abciximab significantly improved coronary flow rates immediately after stenting, which persisted up to 6 months with a significant improvement in residual left ventricular function. The initial bolus dose may also be administered as either an intravenous or intracoronary bolus (Figures 7.5 and 7.6). A meta-analysis by Topol *et al.* showed a significant 30-day mortality benefit with abciximab (Figure 7.7).

The more recent On-TIME 2 study ($n = 984$) compared high-dose tirofiban administered early in the ambulance before primary PCI with placebo. All patients also received aspirin and clopidogrel 600 mg. At 1 year, the tirofiban group had significant lower mortality over placebo.

Except for aspirin, the use of currently available antiplatelet agents (clopidogrel or prasugrel) and anticoagulant agents (unfractionated heparin, enoxaparin, bivalirudin) continues to be evaluated. The recent TRITON-TIMI 38 study showed that prasugrel conferred significant mortality and was superior to clopidogrel in this setting

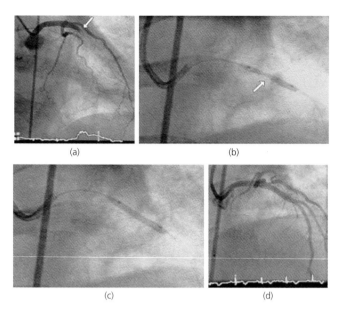

Figure 7.5 Acute anterior ST segment elevation myocardial infarction of 4 hours' duration and severe hypotension, caused by a totally occluded proximal left anterior descending artery (arrow, (a)). After treatment with abciximab, a stent was positioned. Initial inflation showed 'waisting' of the balloon (b), due to fibrous lesion resistance, which resolved on higher inflation (c). Successful recanalisation resulted in brisk flow (d), and the 15-minute procedure completely resolved the patient's chest pain.

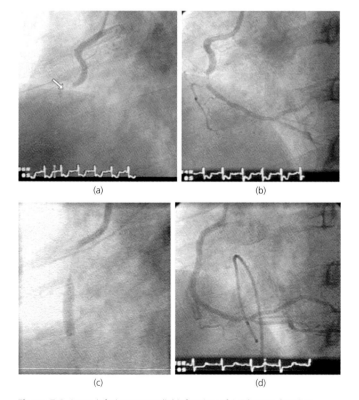

Figure 7.6 Acute inferior myocardial infarction of 2.5 hours' duration caused by a totally occluded middle right coronary artery (arrow, (a)). A guidewire passed through the fresh thrombus produced slow distal filling (b). Deployment of a stent (c) resulted in brisk antegrade flow, a good angiographic result and relief of chest pain (d). A temporary pacemaker electrode was used to counter a reperfusion junctional bradycardia. Note resolution in ST segments compared with top angiograms.

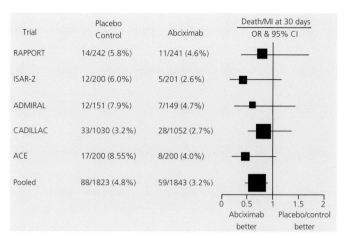

Trial	Placebo Control	Abciximab	Death/MI at 30 days OR & 95% CI
RAPPORT	14/242 (5.8%)	11/241 (4.6%)	
ISAR-2	12/200 (6.0%)	5/201 (2.6%)	
ADMIRAL	12/151 (7.9%)	7/149 (4.7%)	
CADILLAC	33/1030 (3.2%)	28/1052 (2.7%)	
ACE	17/200 (8.55%)	8/200 (4.0%)	
Pooled	88/1823 (4.8%)	59/1843 (3.2%)	

Figure 7.7 Composite 30-day end point of death and myocardial infarction (MI) for five trials of abciximab given before or during primary PCI.

and is currently recommended, except in patients who may be at higher risk of bleeding complications (age >75 years, weight <60 kg, history of previous cerebrovascular events).

Adjunctive mechanical devices

Embolisation of athero-thrombotic material following primary PCI may result in impaired myocardial perfusion. Studies which have evaluated distal protection devices have not been shown to confer significant benefit. In contrast, aspiration catheters significantly improve perfusion and mortality outcomes.

Future of primary PCI

In optimal conditions, primary PCI is the 'gold standard' treatment of acute ST segment elevation myocardial infarction. Where there are practical limitations, the alternatives may be pharmaco-invasive or thrombolytic therapy.

A strategy of primary stenting and thrombus aspiratation, in association with aspirin, heparin, prasugrel (or clopidogrel) and abciximab seems to be the current standard of care, although studies will continue to examine the potential benefit of new antiplatelet and anti-thrombotic agents. The question of whether on-site surgical cover is still essential for infarct intervention continues to be debated.

Further reading

Antman EM, Hand M, Armstrong PW *et al.* 2007 focused update of the ACC/AHA 2004 guidelines for the management of patients with ST-elevation myocardial infarction. A report of the American College of Cardiology/Amercan Heart Association task force on practice guidelines. *J Am Coll Cardiol* 2008;**51**:210–47.

Brar SS, Leon MB, Stone GW *et al.* Use of drug-eluting stents in acute myocardial infarction. *J Am Coll Cardiol* 2009;**53**:1677–89.

De Boer MJ, Zijlstra E. Coronary angioplasty in acute myocardial infarction. In: Grech ED, Ramsdale DR, eds. *Practical Interventional Cardiology*. 2nd ed. London: Martin Dunitz, 2002:189–206.

Fibrinolytic Therapy Trialists' (FIT) Collaborative Group. Indications for fibrinolytic therapy in suspected acute myocardial infarction: collaborative overview of early mortality and major morbidity results from all randomised trials of more than 1000 patients. *Lancet* 1994;**343**:311–22.

Grines CL, Cox DA, Stone GW *et al.*, for the Stent Primary Angioplasty in Myocardial Infarction Study Group. Coronary angioplasty with or without stent implantation for acute myocardial infarction. *N Engl J Med* 1999;**341**:1949–56.

Keeley EC, Boura JA, Grines CL. Primary angioplasty versus intravenous thrombolytic therapy for acute myocardial infarction: a quantitative review of 23 randomised trials. *Lancet* 2003;**361**:13–20.

Stone GW, Grines CL, Cox DA *et al.* Comparison of angioplasty with stenting, with or without abciximab, in acute myocardial infarction. *N Engl J Med* 2002;**346**:957–66.

Topol EJ, Neumann FJ, Montalescot G. A preferred reperfusion strategy for acute myocardial infarction. *J Am Coll Cardiol* 2009;**53**:1677–89.

CHAPTER 8

Percutaneous Coronary Intervention: Cardiogenic Shock

Ever D. Grech

South Yorkshire Cardiothoracic Centre, Northern General Hospital, Sheffield, UK

OVERVIEW

- Cardiogenic shock occurs in 3–7% of acute myocardial infarction hospital admissions and is the commonest cause of early death

- Cardiogenic shock has a very high mortality and the mortality benefit of thrombolytic therapy alone is limited

- Although pharmacological and intra-aortic balloon pump (IABP) support may increase systemic blood pressure, these are temporary and have no effect on long-term survival

- Once cardiogenic shock is recognised (before or after hospital admission), the patient should be urgently transferred to the catheter laboratory

- Pharmacological and IABP support measures, combined with emergency angiography followed by percutaneous coronary intervention (PCI) (or coronary artery bypass graft (CABG)) revascularisation, offer the best survival strategy

---

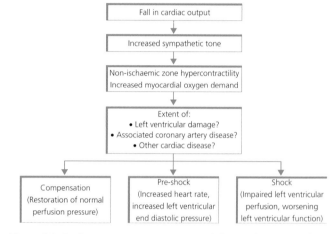

Figure 8.1 Cardiac compensatory response to falling cardiac output after acute myocardial infarction.

Cardiogenic shock is the commonest cause of death after acute myocardial infarction. It occurs in approximately 7% of patients with ST segment elevation myocardial infarction and 3% with non-ST segment elevation myocardial infarction.

Cardiogenic shock is a complex syndrome that involves decreased cardiac output, a progressive state of hypotension (systolic blood pressure <90 mmHg) lasting at least 30 minutes, despite adequate preload and heart rate, which leads to end-organ hypoperfusion. It is usually caused by left ventricular systolic dysfunction. A patient requiring drug or mechanical support to maintain a systolic blood pressure over 90 mmHg can also be considered as manifesting cardiogenic shock. As cardiac output and blood pressure fall, there is an increase in sympathetic tone, with subsequent cardiac and systemic effects, such as altered mental state, cold extremities, peripheral cyanosis and urine output <30 ml/hour.

Effects of cardiogenic shock

Cardiac effects

In an attempt to maintain cardiac output, the remaining non-ischaemic myocardium becomes hypercontractile, and its oxygen consumption increases (Figure 8.1). The effectiveness of this response depends on the extent of current and previous left ventricular damage, the severity of coexisting coronary artery disease and the presence of other cardiac pathology such as valve disease.

Three possible outcomes may occur:

- Compensation – which restores normal blood pressure and myocardial perfusion pressure.
- Partial compensation – which results in a pre-shock state with mildly depressed cardiac output and blood pressure, as well as an elevated heart rate and left ventricular filling pressure.
- Shock – which develops rapidly and leads to profound hypotension and worsening global myocardial ischaemia. Without immediate reperfusion, patients in this group have little potential for myocardial salvage or survival.

Systemic effects

The fall in blood pressure increases catecholamine levels, which in turn leads to systemic arterial and venous constriction. In time, activation of the renin–aldosterone–angiotensin axis causes further vasoconstriction, with subsequent sodium and water retention. These responses have the effect of increasing left ventricular filling pressure and volume. Although this partly compensates for the

ABC of Interventional Cardiology, 2nd edition.
© Ever D. Grech. Published 2011 Blackwell Publishing Ltd.

decline in left ventricular function, a high left ventricular filling pressure leads to pulmonary oedema, which impairs gas exchange. The ensuing respiratory acidosis exacerbates cardiac ischaemia, left ventricular dysfunction and intravascular thrombosis.

Time course of cardiogenic shock

The onset of cardiogenic shock is variable. In patients with acute myocardial infarction recruited into the GUSTO-I study, 7% developed cardiogenic shock – 11% on admission and 89% in the subsequent 2 weeks. Almost all of those who developed cardiogenic shock did so by 48 hours after the onset of symptoms, and their overall 30-day mortality was 57%, compared with an overall study group mortality of just 7%.

Differential diagnosis

Hypotension can complicate acute myocardial infarction in other settings.

Right coronary artery occlusion

An occluded right coronary artery (which usually supplies a smaller proportion of the left ventricular muscle than the left coronary artery) may lead to hypotension in various ways: cardiac output can fall due to vagally mediated reflex venodilatation and bradycardia, and right ventricular dilation may displace the intraventricular septum towards the left ventricular cavity, preventing proper filling.

In addition, the right coronary artery occasionally supplies a sizeable portion of left ventricular myocardium. In this case, right ventricular myocardial infarction produces a unique set of physical findings, haemodynamic characteristics and ST segment elevation in lead V$_4$R (Table 8.1). Predominant right ventricular shock occurs in only 5% of cardiogenic shock cases, but when this occurs, aggressive treatment is indicated as the mortality exceeds 30%.

Ventricular septal defect, mitral regurgitation or myocardial rupture

In 10% of patients with cardiogenic shock, hypotension arises from a ventricular septal defect induced by myocardial infarction or severe mitral regurgitation after papillary muscle rupture. Such a condition should be suspected if a patient develops a new systolic murmur, and is readily confirmed by echocardiography – which should be urgently requested. Such patients have high mortality,

Table 8.1 Hallmarks of right ventricular infarction.

- Rising jugular venous pressure, Kussmaul's sign, pulsus paradoxus
- Low output with little pulmonary congestion
- Right atrial pressure >10 mmHg and >80% of pulmonary capillary wedge pressure
- Right atrial prominent Y descent
- Right ventricle shows dip-and-plateau pattern of pressure
- Profound hypoxia with right to left shunt through a patent foramen ovale
- ST segment elevation in lead V$_4$R

and urgent referral for surgery may be needed. Even with surgery, the survival rate can be low.

Myocardial rupture of the free wall may cause low cardiac output as a result of cardiac compression due to tamponade. It is more difficult to diagnose clinically (raised venous pressure, pulsus paradoxus), but the presence of haemopericardium can be readily confirmed by echocardiography. Pericardial aspiration often leads to rapid increase in cardiac output, and surgery may be necessary.

Miscellaneous

In the absence of the above, other conditions which may present with cardiogenic shock, ST segment elevation and elevated cardiac markers include stress-induced cardiomyopathy (takotsubo cardiomyopathy), acute myopericarditis and hypertrophic cardiomyopathy. Aortic dissection may also result in severe aortic regurgitation, tamponade or myocardial infarction due to coronary occlusion.

Massive pulmonary embolism and severe aortic or mitral disease may also present with cardiogenic shock.

Management

The left ventricular filling volume should be optimised, and in the absence of pulmonary congestion, a saline fluid challenge of at least 250 ml should be administered over 10 minutes. Adequate oxygenation is crucial, and intubation or ventilation should be used early if gas exchange abnormalities are present. Ongoing hypotension induces respiratory muscle failure and this is prevented with mechanical ventilation. Anti-thrombotic treatment (aspirin, clopidogrel and heparin) is appropriate. Drugs which may exacerbate cardiogenic shock (β-blockers, angiotensin-converting enzyme inhibitors, high-dose diuretics) should be avoided.

Supporting systemic blood pressure

Blood pressure support maintains perfusion of vital organs and slows or reverses the metabolic effects of organ hypoperfusion. Inotropes stimulate myocardial function and increase vascular tone, allowing perfusion pressures to increase. Intra-aortic balloon pump counterpulsation often has a dramatic effect on systemic blood pressure (Table 8.2). Inflation occurs in early diastole, greatly increasing aortic diastolic pressure to levels above aortic systolic pressure. In addition, balloon deflation during the start of systole reduces the aortic pressure, thereby decreasing myocardial oxygen demand and forward resistance (afterload) (Figures 8.2–8.5).

Newer supportive percutaneous ventricular assist devices that are being assessed include the TandemHeart and Impella devices (Figure 8.6). These may be used as a bridge to surgery or percutaneous intervention.

Reperfusion

Although inotropic drugs and mechanical support increase systemic blood pressure, these measures are temporary and have no effect on

Table 8.2 Main indications and contraindications for intra-aortic balloon pump counterpulsation.

Indications
- Cardiogenic shock
- Unstable and refractory angina
- Cardiac support for high-risk percutaneous intervention
- Hypoperfusion after coronary artery bypass graft surgery
- Septic shock
- Enhancement of coronary flow after successful recanalisation by percutaneous intervention
- Ventricular septal defect and papillary muscle rupture after myocardial infarction
- Intractable ischaemic ventricular tachycardia

Contraindications
- Severe aortic regurgitation
- Abdominal or aortic aneurysm
- Severe aorto-iliac disease or peripheral vascular disease

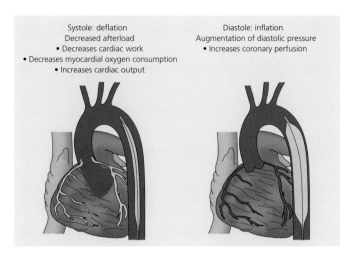

Systole: deflation
Decreased afterload
- Decreases cardiac work
- Decreases myocardial oxygen consumption
- Increases cardiac output

Diastole: inflation
Augmentation of diastolic pressure
- Increases coronary perfusion

Figure 8.3 Effects of intra-aortic balloon pump during systole and diastole.

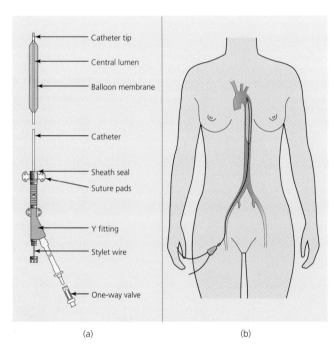

(a)   (b)

Figure 8.2 Diagram of intra-aortic balloon pump (a) and its position in the aorta (b).

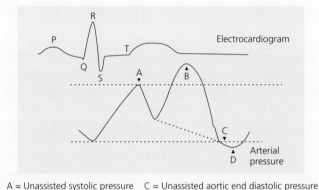

A = Unassisted systolic pressure   C = Unassisted aortic end diastolic pressure
B = Diastolic augmentation   D = Reduced aortic end diastolic pressure

Figure 8.4 Diagram of electrocardiogram and aortic pressure wave showing timing of intra-aortic balloon pump and its effects of diastolic augmentation (D) and reduced aortic end diastolic pressure.

long-term survival unless they are combined with coronary artery recanalisation and myocardial reperfusion (Figure 8.7).

Thrombolysis is currently the commonest form of treatment for acute ST segment elevation myocardial infarction. However, successful fibrinolysis probably depends on drug delivery to the clot, and as blood pressure falls, reperfusion becomes less likely. One study (GISSI) showed that, in patients with cardiogenic shock, streptokinase conferred no benefit compared with placebo.

The GUSTO-I investigators examined data on 2200 patients who either presented with cardiogenic shock or who developed it after enrolment and survived for at least an hour after its onset. Thirty-day mortality was considerably less in those undergoing early angiography (38%) than in patients with late or no

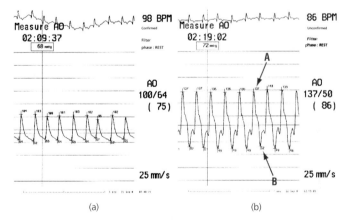

(a)   (b)

Figure 8.5 Aortic pressure wave recording before (a) and during (b) intra-aortic balloon pump counterpulsation in a patient with cardiogenic shock after myocardial infarction. Note marked augmentation in diastolic pressure (arrow A) and reduction in end diastolic pressures (arrow B). (AO, aortic pressure).

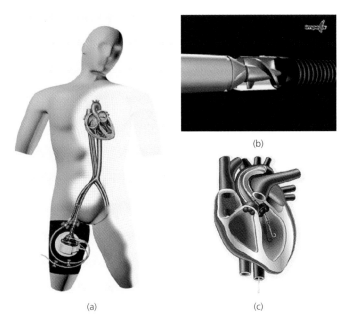

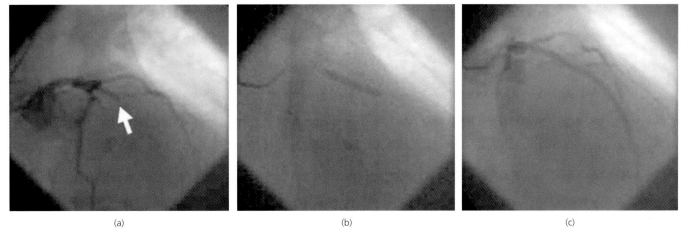

Figure 8.6 (a) The TandemHeart system consists of a low-speed centrifugal continuous flow pump, which is able to deliver up to 4 litres/minute at a rotation of 7500 rpm. Following transeptal puncture, a left atrial cannula removes oxygenated blood, which is returned to the lower abdominal aorta by way of a femoral arterial cannula. (b and c) The Impella device is a small rotary blood pump mounted on a catheter, which is positioned across the aortic valve. Left ventricular blood is aspirated and expelled into the aorta delivering up to 2.5 litres/minute at a rotation of 50 000 rpm.

angiography (62%). Further analysis suggested that early angiography was independently associated with a 43% reduction in 30-day mortality.

In the SHOCK trial, patients with cardiogenic shock were treated aggressively with inotropic drugs, intra-aortic balloon pump counterpulsation and thrombolytic drugs. Patients were also randomised to either coronary angiography plus percutaneous intervention (55%) or bypass surgery (38%) within 6 hours, or medical stabilisation (with revascularisation only permitted after 54 hours). Although the 30-day primary end point did not achieve statistical significance, the death rates progressively diverged, and by 12 months the early revascularisation group showed a significant mortality benefit (55%) compared with the medical stabilisation group (70%). The greatest survival benefit was seen in those aged <75 years and those treated early (<6 hours). Given an absolute risk reduction of 15% at 12 months, one life would be saved for only seven patients treated by aggressive, early revascularisation.

Longer term survival data up to 6 years have shown a persistence of treatment benefit with early revascularisation (41.4% vs 32.8%). These findings are consistent with 55% (11-year survival rate) in the GUSTO-I trial among 30-day cardiogenic shock survivors.

Support and reperfusion: Impact on survival

Over the past 10 years, specific measures to improve blood pressure and restore coronary arterial perfusion have been instituted. Mortality data collected since the 1970s show a significant fall in mortality of 80–90% in the 1990s to the current rate of around 50%. This has been the result of increased use of combinations of thrombolytic drugs, the intra-aortic balloon pump and coronary angiography with revascularisation by either percutaneous intervention or bypass surgery.

Cardiogenic shock is the commonest cause of death in acute myocardial infarction. Although thrombolysis can be attempted with inotropic support or augmentation of blood pressure with the intra-aortic balloon pump, the greatest mortality benefit is seen after urgent coronary angiography and revascularisation, usually PCI. Cardiogenic shock due to acute myocardial infarction is a catheter laboratory emergency.

Figure 8.7 A 65-year old man with a 3–4 hour history of acute anterior myocardial infarction had cardiogenic shock and acute pulmonary oedema, requiring mechanical ventilation and inotropic support. He underwent emergency angiography (a), which showed a totally occluded proximal left anterior descending artery (arrow). A soft tipped guidewire was passed across the occlusive thrombotic lesion, which was successfully stented (b). Restoration of brisk antegrade flow down this artery (c) followed by insertion of an intra-aortic balloon pump markedly improved blood pressure and organ perfusion. The next day he was extubated and weaned off all inotropic drugs, and the intra-aortic balloon pump was removed.

Further reading

Hochman JS, Sleeper LA, Webb JG *et al.* Early revascularization and long-term survival in cardiogenic shock complicating acute myocardial infarction. *J Am Med Assoc* 2006;**295**:2511–15.

Jeger RV, Radovanovic D, Hunziker PR *et al.* Ten-year trends in the incidence and treatment of cardiogenic shock. *Ann Intern Med* 2008;**149**:618–26.

Singh M, White J, Hasdai D *et al.* Long term outcome and its predictors among patients with ST-elevation myocardial infarction complicated by cardiogenic shock: insights from the GUSTO-I trial. *J Am Coll Cardiol* 2007;**50**:1752–8.

White HD. Cardiogenic shock: a more aggressive approach is now warranted. *Eur Heart J* 2000;**21**:1897–901.

CHAPTER 9

Interventional Pharmacotherapy

Ever D. Grech[1] *and Robert F. Storey*[2]

[1] South Yorkshire Cardiothoracic Centre, Northern General Hospital, Sheffield, UK
[2] University of Sheffield, Sheffield, UK

OVERVIEW

- The recent dramatic increase in percutaneous coronary intervention (PCI) has been facilitated by advances in adjunctive pharmacotherapy that have made procedures much safer

- PCI inevitably damages the vessel wall causing platelet and coagulation system activation. This increases the risk of thrombosis at the angioplasty site, as well as distal embolisation, leading to ischaemia and infarction

- Glycoprotein IIb/IIIa inhibitors significantly reduce ischaemic complications during high-risk PCI and have advanced the practice of interventional cardiology especially in the management of acute coronary syndromes

- A combination of aspirin with either clopidogrel or prasugrel has become the mainstay of antiplatelet therapy after stenting to prevent thrombosis within the stent

- Clopidogrel is usually given for 28 days following PCI for chronic stable angina if a bare metal stent is deployed. During this time, a new endothelial lining grows inside the stent, which reduces stent thrombosis

- Clopidogrel or prasugrel is advocated for 12 months in acute coronary syndromes or if a drug-eluting stent is deployed

- Prasugrel may be preferable to clopidogrel in patients undergoing primary PCI for acute ST segment elevation myocardial infarction, in diabetes patients undergoing PCI for any acute coronary syndrome and those who present acutely with stent thrombosis despite clopidogrel therapy

The dramatic increase in the use of percutaneous coronary intervention (PCI) has been possible because of advances in adjunctive pharmacotherapy, which have greatly improved safety and outcomes.

Rupture or erosion of an atherosclerotic plaque or percutaneous coronary intervention – which inevitably causes vessel trauma and disruption of the endothelium and atheromatous plaque – leads to exposure of a thrombogenic surface in the subendothelial layers and release of thrombogenic substances (Figure 9.1). This leads to the recruitment and activation of platelets and the activation of the coagulation cascade, leading to localised thrombosis; this

may impair blood flow, precipitate vessel occlusion or cause distal embolisation. Coronary stents exacerbate this problem as they are thrombogenic. For these reasons, drug inhibition of thrombus formation during PCI is mandatory. However, this must be balanced against the risk of bleeding, both systemic and at the access site.

Coronary artery thrombosis

Platelets are designed to respond rapidly to endothelial damage by adhering to collagen and bound von Willebrand factor and releasing or mediating generation of soluble activators such as adenosine diphosphate (ADP), thromboxane A_2 (TXA_2), 5-hydroxytryptamine (5-HT), adenosine triphosphate (ATP) and thrombin, which lead to the activation of other platelets and their recruitment into an evolving thrombus (Figure 9.2).

Platelets have a large number of glycoprotein IIb/IIIa receptors ($\alpha_{IIb}\beta_3$) and platelet activation converts these receptors to a state of high affinity for fibrinogen, which mediates the cross-linking of platelets and consequent aggregation.

Vascular injury and membrane damage also trigger coagulation by exposure of tissue factor. The resulting thrombin formation further activates platelets and converts fibrinogen to fibrin. Platelets are therefore central to thrombus formation.

Understanding of these mechanisms has led to the development of potent anticoagulants and platelet inhibitors that can be used for PCI (Table 9.1). Since the early days of percutaneous transluminal coronary angioplasty, heparin and aspirin have remained a fundamental part of PCI treatment. Following the introduction of stents, ticlopidine and more recently clopidogrel and prasugrel have allowed a very low rate of stent thrombosis. Glycoprotein IIb/IIIa receptor antagonists have reduced procedural complications still further and improved the protection of the distal microcirculation, especially in thrombus-containing lesions prevalent in acute coronary syndromes.

Bleeding

Major bleeding after PCI is strongly linked with a fivefold increase in late mortality. This risk is dependent not only on patient characteristics (such as advanced age, female gender, renal impairment, diabetes, hypertension and malignancy) but also on the choice

ABC of Interventional Cardiology, 2nd edition.
© Ever D. Grech. Published 2011 Blackwell Publishing Ltd.

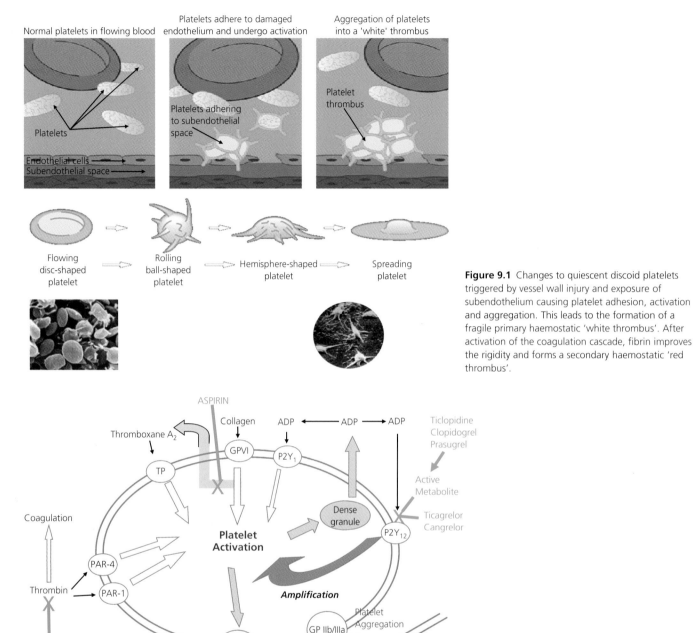

Figure 9.1 Changes to quiescent discoid platelets triggered by vessel wall injury and exposure of subendothelium causing platelet adhesion, activation and aggregation. This leads to the formation of a fragile primary haemostatic 'white thrombus'. After activation of the coagulation cascade, fibrin improves the rigidity and forms a secondary haemostatic 'red thrombus'.

Figure 9.2 Targets for platelet inhibition. GP, glycoprotein; PAR, protease-activated receptor; TP, thromboxane A_2/prostaglandin H_2.

of vascular access (higher in femoral than radial) and the choice of anti-thrombotic regimen. Irrespective of any previous cardiac procedure, advanced age and some co-morbidities such as renal failure are associated with higher mortality. Also, intracranial or gastrointestinal bleeds are well recognised as potentially fatal events. However, other mechanisms linking bleeding (and blood transfusion) after PCI with excess mortality have been difficult to identify and require further study. Efforts continue to be made to identify new anti-thrombotic approaches capable of reducing bleeding complications whilst retaining an equivalent anti-ischaemic profile.

Anticoagulant drugs

Unfractionated heparin and low molecular weight heparin

Unfractionated heparin is a heterogeneous mucopolysaccharide that binds antithrombin, which greatly potentiates the inhibition of thrombin, and factor Xa (Figure 9.3). It has been the traditional choice of anticoagulant for reducing the risk of coronary artery and catheter thrombosis. Its very low cost and relatively short half-life, the ability to rapidly reverse its effects with protamine

Table 9.1 Adjunctive pharmacology during percutaneous coronary intervention.

Aspirin – for all clinical settings
Clopidogrel/Prasugrel – for stenting; chronic stable angina, unstable angina, non-ST segment elevation myocardial infarction and ST segment elevation myocardial infarction
Unfractionated and low molecular weight heparin – for all clinical settings
Fondaparinux – for medical management of acute coronary syndromes prior to PCI
Glycoprotein IIb/IIIa receptor inhibitors

  Abciximab – for elective percutaneous intervention for chronic stable angina; unstable angina or non-ST segment elevation myocardial infarction (before and during percutaneous intervention); ST segment elevation myocardial infarction (before and during primary percutaneous intervention)
  Eptifibatide – for elective percutaneous intervention for chronic stable angina; unstable angina or non-ST segment elevation myocardial infarction (before and during percutaneous intervention)
  Tirofiban – for unstable angina or non-ST segment elevation myocardial infarction (before and during percutaneous intervention)

and the availability of assays to monitor its anticoagulant effect are advantages (Table 9.2). However, an important limitation of unfractionated heparin is its unpredictable anticoagulant effect due to variable, non-specific binding to plasma proteins. Side effects include haemorrhage at the access site and heparin-induced thrombocytopenia. About 10–20% of patients may develop type-I thrombocytopenia, which is usually mild and self-limiting. About 0.3–3.0% of patients exposed to heparin for longer than 5 days develop the more serious immune-mediated, type-II thrombocytopenia, which paradoxically, may be associated with thrombosis by platelet activation. However, this complication is unlikely when heparin is used just to cover the PCI procedure.

Enoxaparin, a low molecular weight heparin, and fondaparinux, a synthetic factor Xa antagonist, have less or no prothrombotic effect, are longer acting and have more consistent response than unfractionated heparin. Enoxaparin is only partially reversible with protamine. Enoxaparin and fondaparinux are administered by subcutaneous or intravenous injection and are frequently used in the setting of non-ST segment elevation acute coronary syndromes prior to coronary angiography. They may also be of particular benefit when administered intravenously at the time of PCI and further studies are planned to compare these anticoagulants in this setting. For patients already taking a therapeutic dose of low molecular weight heparin who need urgent PCI, a switch to unfractionated heparin may not be necessary if the last dose was given less than 8 hours before the PCI.

Direct thrombin inhibitors

These include hirudin, bivalirudin, lepirudin and argatroban. They directly bind thrombin and act independently of antithrombin III. They bind less to plasma proteins and have a more predictable dose response than unfractionated heparin. Bivalirudin is the most commonly used and studies have shown that it has similar medium-term rates of ischaemic events and less bleeding compared to the combination of unfractionated heparin with a glycoprotein IIb/IIIa

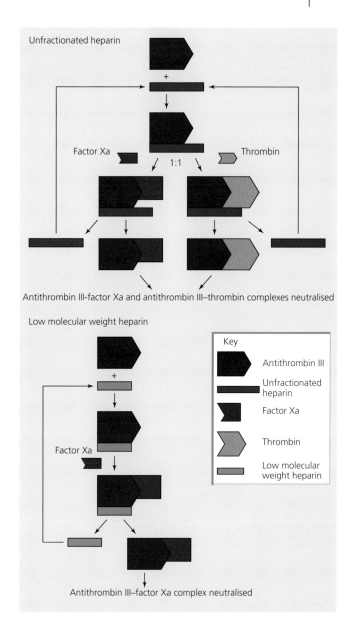

Figure 9.3 Mechanisms of catalytic inhibitory action of unfractionated heparin and low molecular weight heparin. Unfractionated heparin interacts with antithrombin III, accelerating binding and neutralisation of thrombin and factor Xa (in 1:1 ratio). Dissociated heparin is then free to rebind with antithrombin III. Low molecular weight heparin is less able to bind thrombin because of its shorter length. This results in selective inactivation of factor Xa relative to thrombin. Irreversibly bound antithrombin III and factor Xa complex is neutralised, and dissociated low molecular weight heparin is free to rebind with antithrombin III.

receptor antagonist in patients undergoing PCI for acute coronary syndromes. Bivalirudin may also be used in patients with immune-mediated, heparin-induced thrombocytopenia.

Antiplatelet drugs

Aspirin

Aspirin (acetylsalicylic acid) irreversibly inhibits cyclooxygenase in platelets, preventing the synthesis and release of prothrombotic

Table 9.2 Comparison of unfractionated heparin and low molecular weight heparin.

Unfractionated heparin	Low molecular weight heparin
Molecular weight: 3000–30 000 Da	*Molecular weight*: 4000–6000 Da
Mechanism of action: binds antithrombin and inactivates factor Xa and thrombin equally (1:1)	*Mechanism of action*: binds antithrombin and inactivates factor Xa more than thrombin (2–4:1)
Pharmacokinetics: variable binding to plasma proteins, endothelial cells and macrophages, giving unpredictable anticoagulant effects	*Pharmacokinetics*: minimal plasma protein binding and no binding to endothelial cells and macrophages, giving predictable anticoagulant effects
Short half-life	Longer half-life
Reversible with protamine	Partially reversible with protamine
Laboratory monitoring: activated clotting time	*Laboratory monitoring*: not required
Cost: inexpensive	*Cost*: 10–20 times more expensive than unfractionated heparin

thromboxane-A2 during platelet activation. Aspirin given before percutaneous intervention reduces the risk of abrupt arterial closure by 50–75%. It is well tolerated, with a low incidence of serious adverse effects (gastric erosion and haemorrhage). The standard dose results in full effect within hours, and in patients with established coronary artery disease it is given indefinitely. However, aspirin is only a mild antiplatelet agent and the risk of acute stent thrombosis is relatively high if aspirin is the only oral antiplatelet agent administered. These drawbacks have led to the development of another class of antiplatelet drugs, the thienopyridines.

Thienopyridines

Ticlopidine, clopidogrel and prasugrel belong to the thienopyridine class of oral antiplatelet agents. These are converted by hepatic cytochrome P450 (CYP) enzymes into active metabolites that bind irreversibly to the platelet ADP receptors designated $P2Y_{12}$ and consequently prevent activation of this receptor by ADP.

The combination of aspirin with clopidogrel or prasugrel has become a standard antiplatelet treatment during stenting in order to prevent thrombosis within the stent. Ticlopidine is no longer in common clinical use because of its side-effect profile.

The loading dose of clopidogrel is 600 mg at the time of stenting or 75 mg daily at least 5 days beforehand. In patients undergoing bare metal stent PCI for chronic stable angina, it is continued for about 4 weeks, until new endothelium covers the inside of the stent. However, the CURE and CREDO studies support the much longer term (1 year) use of clopidogrel and aspirin after PCI, having found a significant (27%) reduction in combined risk of death, myocardial infarction or stroke. In addition, longer term administration of clopidogrel (at least 1 year) is also recommended in patients undergoing drug-eluting stent PCI in view of the delayed stent endothelialisation and higher risk of late stent thrombosis.

There is a substantial inter-individual variability in the pharmacodynamic response to clopidogrel mediated in part by variations in the gene for CYP2C19, age, weight, co-medication that inhibits relevant CYP enzymes (such as omeprazole) and certain disease states.

Patients with poor pharmacodynamic response to clopidogrel are at greater risk of ischaemic events. Prasugrel is more potent with more rapid, consistent and predictable antiplatelet response. Consequently, it was shown in the TRITON-TIMI 38 study to have superior efficacy than clopidogrel in patients undergoing PCI for non-ST segment elevation and ST segment elevation acute coronary syndromes, although it also significantly increased rates of major and fatal haemorrhage. This was particularly evident in elderly patients ≥75 years, patients with a body weight <60 kg and those with a history of cerebrovascular event. Current guidelines recommend prasugrel in patients undergoing primary PCI for acute ST segment elevation myocardial infarction, in diabetes patients undergoing PCI for any acute coronary syndrome and those who present acutely with stent thrombosis whilst taking clopidogrel. The loading dose of prasugrel is 60 mg followed by a 10-mg daily maintenance dose for 1 year. A reduced daily dose of 5 mg is recommended for those with a body weight <60 kg or those aged ≥75 years, although the use of prasugrel is cautioned in the latter group. Prasugrel is contraindicated in patients with a history of a cerebrovascular event or at high risk of bleeding.

Reversibly acting, non-thienopyridine $P2Y_{12}$ antagonists, such as ticagrelor and cangrelor, are being assessed. The recent PLATO study demonstrated that ticagrelor was superior to clopidogrel including a significant reduction in mortality, without an overall cost in bleeding. Cangrelor, an intravenous $P2Y_{12}$ antagonist has also been compared with clopidogrel in the two CHAMPION studies. Whilst cangrelor did inhibit platelet activity more effectively than clopidogrel, this did not translate into a reduction of the primary end points of death, myocardial infarction and ischaemia-driven revascularisation at 48 hours.

Glycoprotein IIb/IIIa receptor antagonists

These are potent inhibitors of platelet aggregation (Figure 9.4). The three drugs that are in clinical use are abciximab, eptifibatide and tirofiban (Table 9.3). Abciximab is a monoclonal antibody that binds with high avidity to the glycoprotein IIb/IIIa receptor. It is administered intravenously with slow offset of effect over 24 hours

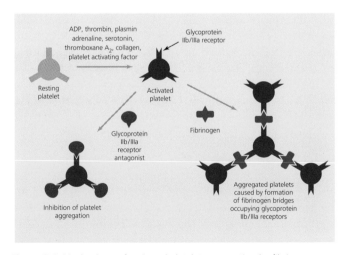

Figure 9.4 Mechanisms of activated platelet aggregation by fibrin cross-linking and its blockade with glycoprotein IIb/IIIa inhibitors.

Table 9.3 Glycoprotein IIb/IIIa inhibitors currently in use.

	Abciximab	Eptifibatide	Tirofiban
Source	Chimeric (humanised) monoclonal mouse antibody	Peptide	Non-peptide
Time for platelet inhibition to return to normal (hours)	24–48	4–6	4–8
Severe thrombocytopenia	1.0% (higher if readministered)	Similar to placebo	Similar to placebo
Reversible with platelet transfusion?	Yes	No	No

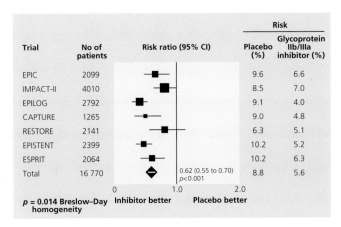

Figure 9.6 Composite 30-day end point of death and myocardial infarction for seven trials of glycoprotein IIb/IIIa inhibitors given before or during planned percutaneous coronary intervention for unstable angina and non-ST segment elevation myocardial infarction.

following cessation of infusion. Eptifibatide and tirofiban are non-antibody ('small molecule'), intravenous glycoprotein IIb/IIIa antagonists that are used as alternatives to abciximab, being cheaper and carrying less risk of the uncommon side effect of severe thrombocytopenia.

Current use of glycoprotein IIb/IIIa receptor antagonists

Elective PCI for chronic stable angina

Although large trials had previously established the benefit of abciximab and eptifibatide (EPISTENT and ESPRIT respectively) in elective PCI for chronic stable angina, these predated the CREDO study, which assessed preloaded clopidogrel prior to PCI which was continued for 1 year. This has led to a reduced global usage of glycoprotein IIb/IIIa receptor antagonists, which are now reserved for those at high risk of thrombotic events or bailout for complications.

Non-ST segment elevation acute coronary syndrome

The current role of glycoprotein IIb/IIIa inhibitors in non-ST segment elevation acute coronary syndrome has been defined by results from several randomised trials. In one meta-analysis, 29,885 patients (largely treated without percutaneous intervention) were randomised to receive a glycoprotein IIb/IIIa inhibitor or placebo

(Figure 9.5). The end point of '30-day death or non-fatal myocardial infarction' showed an overall significant benefit of the glycoprotein IIb/IIIa inhibitor over placebo. Surprisingly, the largest trial (GUSTO IV ACS) showed no benefit with abciximab, which may be partly due to inclusion of lower risk patients. The use of glycoprotein IIb/IIIa inhibitors in all patients with unstable angina and non-ST segment elevation myocardial infarction remains debatable, although the consistent benefit seen with these drugs has led to the recommendation that they be given only to higher risk patients scheduled for PCI.

In another meta-analysis ($n = 16,770$), patients were given a glycoprotein IIb/IIIa inhibitor or placebo immediately before or during planned percutaneous intervention. All showed unequivocal benefit with the active drug (Figure 9.6). The more recent ISAR-REACT 2 study showed that abciximab significantly reduced the risk of adverse events (specifically recurrent myocardial infarction) in those with an elevated troponin level even after pretreatment with 600 mg of clopidogrel. Despite their efficacy, however, some interventionists are reluctant to use glycoprotein IIb/IIIa inhibitors in all patients because of their bleeding risk and reserve their use for high-risk lesions or when complications occur.

ST segment elevation myocardial infarction

In many centres, primary percutaneous intervention is the preferred method of revascularisation for acute myocardial infarction. To date, randomised studies have shown that abciximab or high-dose tirofiban demonstrates benefit in this setting. The development of lower cost alternatives may increase the use of glycoprotein IIb/IIIa inhibitors.

Restenosis

Although coronary stents reduce restenosis rates compared with balloon angioplasty alone, restenosis within stents remains a problem. Whilst anti-thrombotic drugs may reduce the risk of restenosis, nearly all systemic drugs aimed at reducing restenosis have failed, and drug-eluting stents delivering cytotoxic/cytostatic drugs locally

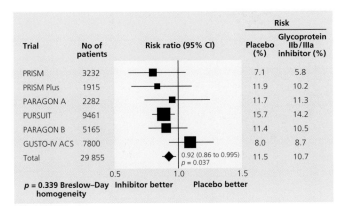

Figure 9.5 Composite 30-day end point of death and myocardial infarction for six medical treatment trials of glycoprotein IIb/IIIa inhibitors in unstable angina and non-ST segment elevation myocardial infarction.

remain the most effective way of preventing restenosis and may ultimately provide the solution to this problem.

The future

Improvements in adjunctive pharmacotherapy, in combination with changes in device technology, will allow PCI to be performed with increased likelihood of acute and long-term success and with lower procedural risks in a wider variety of clinical situations. Further refinements in antiplatelet treatment may soon occur with rapidly available bedside assays to monitor the extent of $P2Y_{12}$ inhibition in patients receiving thienopyridines. The development of new strategies in $P2Y_{12}$ antagonism is likely to lead to a new phase of individualised pharmacotherapy allowing an advanced balance in the risk of ischaemic events and bleeding.

Further reading

Boersma E, Harrington RA, Moliterno DJ et al. Platelet glycoprotein IIb/IIIa inhibitors in acute coronary syndromes: a meta-analysis of all major randomized clinical trials. *Lancet* 2002;**359**:189–98.

Chew DP, Lincoff AM. Adjunctive pharmacotherapy and coronary intervention. In: Grech ED, Ramsdale DR, eds. *Practical Interventional Cardiology*. 2nd ed. London: Martin Dunitz, 2002:207–24.

ESPRIT Investigators. Novel dosing regimen of eptifibatide in planned coronary stent implantation (ESPRIT): a randomized, placebo-controlled trial. *Lancet* 2000;**356**:2037–44.

Lincoff AM, Califf RM, Moliterno DJ et al. Complementary clinical benefits of coronary-artery stenting and blockade of platelet glycoprotein IIb/IIIa receptors. *N Engl J Med* 1999;**341**:319–27.

PRISM-PLUS Study Investigators. Inhibition of the platelet glycoprotein IIb/IIIa receptor with tirofiban in unstable angina and non-Q wave myocardial infarction. Platelet receptor inhibition in ischemic syndrome management in patients limited by unstable signs and symptoms. *N Engl J Med* 1998;**338**:1488–97.

PURSUIT Trial Investigators. Inhibition of platelet glycoprotein IIb/IIIa with eptifibatide in patients with acute coronary syndromes. Platelet glycoprotein IIb/IIIa in unstable angina: receptor suppression using integrilin therapy. *N Engl J Med* 1998;**339**:436–43.

Steinhubl SR, Berger PB, Mann JT 3rd et al. Early and sustained dual oral antiplatelet therapy following percutaneous coronary intervention. A randomized controlled trial. *JAMA* 2002;**288**:2411–20.

Storey RF. New developments in antiplatelet therapy. *Eur Heart J* 2008;**10** (Suppl J):D30–37.

Wallentin L, Becker RC, Budaj A et al. Ticagrelor versus clopidogrel in patients with acute coronary syndromes. *N Engl J Med* 2009;**361**: 1045–57.

Wiviott SD, Braunwald E, McCabe CH et al. Prasugrel versus clopidogrel in patients with acute coronary syndromes. *N Engl J Med* 2007;**357**: 2001–15.

CHAPTER 10

Non-coronary Percutaneous Intervention

Ever D. Grech

South Yorkshire Cardiothoracic Centre, Northern General Hospital, Sheffield, UK

OVERVIEW

- Significant developments in non-coronary, transcatheter cardiac procedures now offer selected patients alternative and less invasive treatments

- Balloon mitral valvuloplasty is the procedure of choice for patients with symptomatic mitral stenosis and suitable valvular anatomy

- Percutaneous mitral valve repair and transcatheter aortic valve implantation (TAVI) are promising new procedures that may be suitable for patients who are at high risk of undergoing conventional cardiac surgery

- Ethanol septal ablation offers symptomatic hypertrophic obstructive cardiomyopathy (HOCM) patients an alternative to myectomy, with a comparable procedural mortality and morbidity and reduction in left ventricular outflow tract (LVOT) gradient

- Percutaneous septal occlusion devices are becoming increasingly used in adults with atrial septal defects (ASDs) and patent foramen ovale (PFOs). Their use in post-myocardial infarction ventricular septal defects (VSDs) is uncertain, but may be considered

Although most percutaneous interventional procedures involve the coronary arteries, major developments in non-coronary transcatheter cardiac procedures have occurred in the past 20 years. In adults, the commonest procedures are balloon mitral valvuloplasty, ethanol septal ablation and septal defect closure. These problems were once treatable only by surgery, but selected patients may now be offered less invasive alternatives. Carrying out such transcatheter procedures require supplementary training to that for coronary intervention.

Balloon mitral valvuloplasty

Acquired mitral stenosis is a consequence of rheumatic fever and is the commonest in developing countries. Commissural fusion, thickening and calcification of the mitral valve leaflets typically occur, as well as thickening and shortening of the chordae tendinae (Figure 10.1). The mitral valve stenosis leads to left atrial

ABC of Interventional Cardiology, 2nd edition.

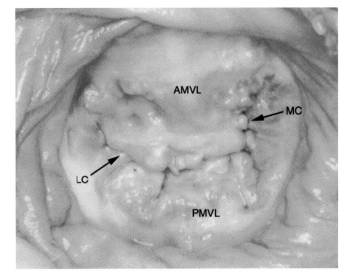

Figure 10.1 Rheumatic chronic mitral valve stenosis showing distorted, fused and calcified valve leaflets. AMVL, anterior mitral valve leaflet; PMVL, posterior mitral valve leaflet; LC, lateral commissure; MC, medial commissure.

enlargement, which predisposes patients to atrial fibrillation and the formation of left atrial thrombus.

In the 1980s, percutaneous balloon valvuloplasty techniques were developed that could open the fused mitral commissures in a manner similar to surgical commissurotomy. The resulting fall in pressure gradient and increase in mitral valve area led to symptomatic improvement. Today, this procedure is most often performed with the hourglass-shaped Inoue balloon. This is introduced into the right atrium from the femoral vein, passed across the atrial septum by way of a septal puncture and then positioned across the stenosed mitral valve before inflation (Figure 10.2).

Patient selection

In general, patients with moderate or severe mitral stenosis (valve area <1.5 cm^2) with symptomatic disease despite optimal medical treatment can be considered for this procedure. Further patient selection relies heavily on transthoracic and transoesophageal echocardiographic findings, which provide structural information about the mitral valve and subvalvar apparatus.

A scoring system for predicting outcomes is commonly used to screen potential candidates. Four characteristics (valve mobility,

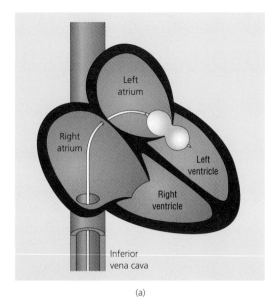

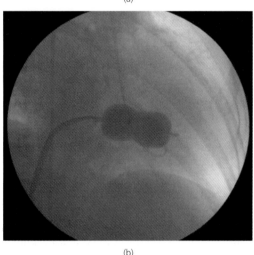

(b)

Figure 10.2 (a) Diagram of the Inoue balloon catheter positioned across a stenosed mitral valve. (b) Fluoroscopic image of the inflated Inoue balloon across the valve.

leaflet thickening, subvalvar thickening and calcification) are each graded from 1 to 4. Patients with a score of <8 are more likely to have a good result than those with scores of >8. Thus, patients with pliable, non-calcified valves and minimal fusion of the subvalvar apparatus achieve the best immediate and long-term results.

Relative contraindications

Relative contraindications are the presence of pre-existing significant mitral regurgitation and left atrial thrombus. Successful balloon valvuloplasty increases valve area to >1.5 cm^2 without a substantial increase in mitral regurgitation, resulting in significant symptomatic improvement.

Complications

The major procedural complications are death (1%), haemopericardium (usually during trans-septal catheterisation, 1%), cerebrovascular embolisation (1%), severe mitral regurgitation (due to a torn valve cusp, 2%) and atrial septal defect (at the transeptal puncture site, although this closes or decreases in size in most patients, 10%). Immediate and long-term results are similar to those with surgical valvotomy, and balloon valvuloplasty can be repeated if commissural restenosis (a gradual process with an incidence of 30–40% at 6–8 years) occurs.

In patients with suitable valvar anatomy, balloon valvuloplasty has become the treatment of choice for mitral stenosis, delaying the need for surgical intervention. It may also be of particular use in those patients who are at high risk of surgical intervention (because of pregnancy, age or coexisting pulmonary or renal disease).

Percutaneous mitral valve repair

Mitral regurgitation often occurs when the two mitral valve leaflets fail to meet correctly (poor coaptation) during ventricular systole and there are two main causes for this. The first is structural abnormality of valve leaflets (usually degenerative), annulus or subvalvular apparatus, resulting in a flail, billowing or prolapsing leaflet. The second, more common cause is left ventricular dilatation, which in turn dilates the mitral annulus resulting in poor leaflet coaptation and disruption of the intricate dynamics of mitral valve function. This is referred to as *functional mitral regurgitation*. The mitral leaflets themselves may appear normal. Other less common causes of regurgitation include valve infection and leaflet erosion (often the result of endocarditis) and rheumatic heart disease.

Long-standing, severe mitral regurgitation leads to progressive left ventricular volume overload and failure, as well as pulmonary hypertension. Myocardial dysfunction may become irreversible due to chronic volume overload. Although diuretic and vasodilator therapies may offer symptomatic relief, they have not been shown to be useful in delaying surgery or improving survival. Patients with moderate to severe (grade 3 or 4) mitral regurgitation who are symptomatic (or if asymptomatic but with evidence of ventricular dysfunction) should be treated by either mitral valve repair or replacement surgery where possible.

However, if the surgical risk is high, advances in technique and equipment have recently facilitated development of methods to treat this via a percutaneous route. These approaches are modifications of established surgical therapies, such as mitral leaflet repair and annuloplasty.

The first is the 24F Mitraclip system (Figure 10.3), which is oriented perpendicular to the line of coaptation, advanced in the left ventricular chamber and deployed by capturing the anterior and posterior mitral valve leaflets simultaneously creating a point of permanent coaptation and a double orifice (Figure 10.4). The barbed gripping element allows capture of the leaflets within the clip arms. If suboptimal results are achieved in the initial attempt, the clip can be reopened, the leaflets released, the clip repositioned and the mitral leaflets regrasped at a different location. Following the encouraging results of preliminary pilot EVEREST 1 study, the EVEREST 2 study had a high-risk registry arm and a randomised arm (MitraClip device or surgical valve replacement in a 2:1 ratio in 279 patients with 3+ to 4+ mitral

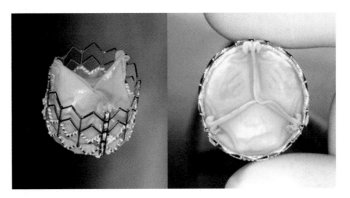

Figure 10.5 The Sapien valve.

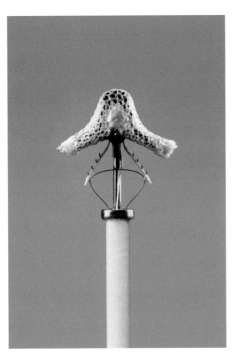

Figure 10.3 The Mitraclip device.

regurgitation). Although the MitraClip was not as good as surgery at reducing mitral regurgitation, the clinical outcomes (NYHA class, quality-of-life surveys) as well as improvements in left ventricular volume and dimensions were similar between the two groups at one year. Interestingly, there were no differences in outcome between the degenerative mitral regurgitation patients and those with functional mitral regurgitation.

In an attempt to mimic the surgical annuloplasty ring, new percutaneous devices are undergoing evaluation but to date none are available for routine clinical use. These include devices that are positioned in the coronary sinus encircling the perimeter of the mitral annulus, with the aim of constricting its circumference to significantly improve the regurgitation.

Transcatheter aortic valve implantation (TAVI)

Aortic stenosis is most often due to calcification of a congenitally bicuspid or normal trileaflet valve. It is the most prevalent

valvular heart disease in developed countries and its prevalence increases with advancing age. Nearly 5% of those over 75% years have moderate or severe aortic stenosis. If symptomatic (angina, syncope or dyspnoea), or if ventricular function is impaired, the prognosis is poor, with an annual mortality of 25%. Furthermore, operative mortality increases with advanced age and approximately one-third of patients with symptomatic aortic stenosis are deemed unsuitable for surgical aortic valve replacement. The development of transcatheter aortic valve implantation (TAVI) has therefore become an attractive option for such patients.

There are currently two available transcatheter valve systems, with others in development. The Sapien valve (Figure 10.5) is a trileaflet bovine pericardium valve mounted on a balloon-expandable stent placed in the subcoronary position. It is introduced via a femoral arterial 22F or 24F sheath, which requires a surgical cut-down procedure. It may also be surgically introduced via the left ventricular transapical route in patients with poor ilio-femoral arterial access. The Corevalve (Figure 10.6) is a trileaflet porcine pericardium valve mounted on a self-expanding nitinol frame. It has a smaller 18F delivery sheath, and a surgical femoral arterial cut-down is not necessary.

Experience in the use of TAVI in suitable patients who are identified as being at high surgical risk (usually defined as having a logistic EuroScore ≥20% or an STS score of ≥10%) is increasing rapidly. A number of ongoing registries involving both the Sapien valve and Corevalve have shown high procedural success rates of around 90%, a stroke rate of around 5% and a 30-day mortality of around 10% – although the apical route mortality is higher. Randomised studies comparing surgery with TAVI are also underway.

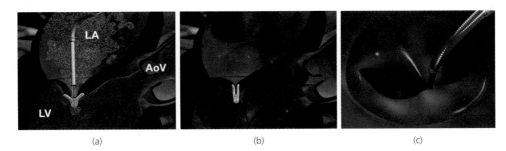

(a) (b) (c)

Figure 10.4 (a) The Mitraclip device simultaneously capturing the anterior and posterior mitral valve leaflets (LA, left atrium; LV, left ventricle; AoV, aortic valve). (b) Deployed device is released showing position of clip on the mitral valve. (c) Point of permanent coaptation and a double orifice, as viewed from the left atrium.

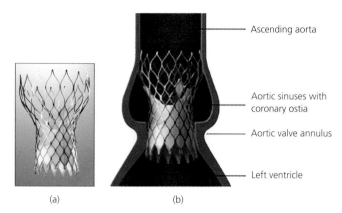

Ascending aorta

Aortic sinuses with coronary ostia

Aortic valve annulus

Left ventricle

(a)   (b)

Figure 10.6 The Corevalve (a) and its deployed position in the aortic root (b).

It is likely that equipment improvements and procedural expertise will increase procedural safety. Whether TAVI will replace surgical valve replacements in younger or lower risk patients is debatable.

Ethanol septal ablation

Hypertrophic cardiomyopathy

Hypertrophic cardiomyopathy is a disease of the myocytes (Figure 10.7) caused by mutations in any one of 10 genes encoding various components of the sarcomeres. It is the commonest genetic cardiovascular disease, being inherited as an autosomal dominant trait and affecting about 1 in 500 of the population. It has highly variable clinical and pathological presentations (Table 10.1).

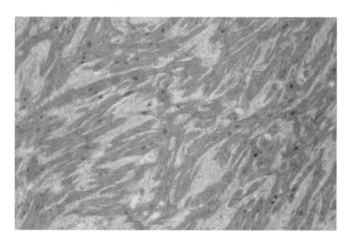

Figure 10.7 Micrograph of hypertrophied myocytes in haphazard alignments characteristic of hypertrophic cardiomyopathy. Interstitial collagen is also increased.

Table 10.1 Characteristics of hypertrophic cardiomyopathy.

Anatomical – ventricular hypertrophy of unknown cause, usually with disproportionate involvement of the interventricular septum
Physiological – well-preserved systolic ventricular function, impaired diastolic relaxation
Pathological – extensive disarray and disorganisation of cardiac myocytes and increased interstitial collagen

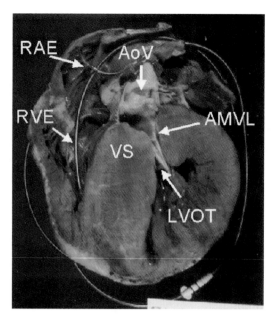

Figure 10.8 Post-mortem appearance of a heart with hypertrophic cardiomyopathy showing massive ventricular and septal hypertrophy causing obstruction of the left ventricular outflow tract (LVOT). This is compounded by the anterior mitral valve leaflet (AMVL), which presses against the ventricular septum (VS). Note the coincidental right atrial (RAE) and right ventricular (RVE) pacing electrodes. AoV, aortic valve.

It is usually diagnosed by echocardiography and is characterised by the presence of unexplained hypertrophy in a non-dilated left ventricle (Figure 10.8). In a quarter of cases, septal enlargement may result in substantial obstruction of the left ventricular outflow tract. This is compounded by Venturi suction movement of the anterior mitral valve leaflet during ventricular systole, bringing it into contact with the hypertrophied septum. The systolic anterior

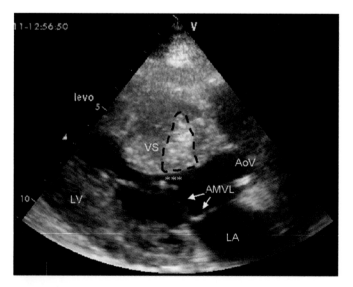

Figure 10.9 Echocardiogram showing anterior mitral valve leaflet (AMVL) and septal contact (***) during ventricular systole. Note marked left ventricular (LV) free wall and ventricular septal (VS) hypertrophy. Injection of an echocontrast agent down the septal artery results in an area of septal echo-brightness (dotted line). LA, left atrium; AoV, aortic valve.

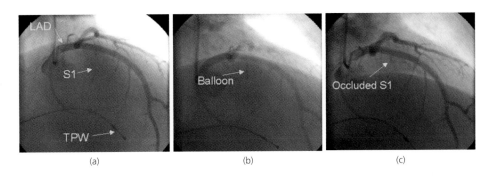

Figure 10.10 Angiograms showing ethanol septal ablation. The first septal artery (S1, (a)) is occluded with a balloon catheter (b) before ethanol injection. This results in permanent septal artery occlusion (c) and a localised septal myocardial infarction. LAD, left anterior descending artery; TPW, temporary pacemaker wire.

motion (SAM) of the anterior mitral valve leaflet also causes mitral regurgitation.

Treatment

Although hypertrophic cardiomyopathy is often asymptomatic, common symptoms are dyspnoea, angina and exertional syncope, which may be related to the gradient in the left ventricular outflow tract. The aim of treatment of symptomatic patients is to improve functional disability, reduce the extent of obstruction of the left ventricular outflow tract and improve diastolic filling. Treatments include negatively inotropic drugs such as β-blockers, verapamil and disopyramide. However, 10% of symptomatic patients fail to respond to drugs, and surgery – ventricular myectomy (which usually involves removal of a small amount of septal muscle) or ethanol septal ablation – can be considered.

The objective of ethanol septal ablation is to induce a localised septal myocardial infarction at the site of obstruction of the left ventricular outflow tract. The procedure involves threading a small balloon catheter into the septal artery supplying the culprit area of septum. Echocardiography with injection of an echocontrast agent down the septal artery allows the appropriate septal artery to be identified and reduces the number of unnecessary ethanol injections (Figure 10.9).

Once the appropriate artery is identified, the catheter balloon is inflated to completely occlude the vessel, and a small amount of dehydrated ethanol is injected through the central lumen of the catheter into the distal septal artery. This causes immediate and permanent vessel occlusion and localised myocardial infarction (Figure 10.10). The infarct reduces septal motion and thickness, enlarges the left ventricular outflow tract, and may decrease mitral valve systolic anterior motion, with consequent reduction in the gradient of the left ventricular outflow tract (Figure 10.11) and decrease in the degree of mitral regurgitation. Over the next few months, the infarcted septum undergoes fibrosis and shrinkage, which may result in further symptomatic improvement.

The procedure is performed under local anaesthesia with sedation as required. Patients inevitably experience chest discomfort during ethanol injection, and treatment with intravenous opiate analgesics is essential. Patients are usually discharged after 4 or 5 days.

Complications

Heart block is a frequent acute complication, so a temporary pacing electrode is inserted via the femoral vein beforehand and is usually left in situ for 24 hours after the procedure, during which time the patient is monitored.

The main procedural complications are persistent heart block requiring a permanent pacemaker (10%), coronary artery dissection and infarction requiring immediate coronary artery bypass grafting (2%) and death (1–2%). The procedural mortality and morbidity is similar to that for surgical myectomy, as is the

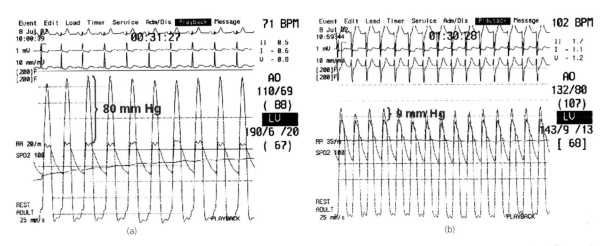

Figure 10.11 Simultaneous aortic and left ventricular pressure waves before (a) and after (b) successful ethanol septal ablation. Note the difference between left ventricular peak pressure and aortic peak pressure, which represents the left ventricular outflow tract gradient, has been reduced from 80 mmHg to 9 mmHg. BPM, beats per minute, AO, aorta .

reduction in left ventricular outflow tract gradient. Surgery and ethanol septal ablation have not as yet been directly compared in randomised studies.

Septal defect closure

Atrial septal defects

Atrial septal defects are congenital abnormalities characterised by a structural deficiency of the atrial septum and account for about 10% of all congenital cardiac disease. The commonest atrial septal defects affect the ostium secundum (in the fossa ovalis), and most are suitable for transcatheter closure. Although atrial septal defects may be closed in childhood, they are the commonest form of congenital heart disease to become apparent in adulthood.

Diagnosis is usually confirmed by echocardiography, allowing visualisation of the anatomy of the defect and Doppler estimation of the shunt size. The physiological importance of the defect depends on the duration and size of the shunt, as well as the response of the pulmonary vascular bed. Patients with significant shunts (defined as a ratio of pulmonary blood flow to systemic blood flow >1.5) should be considered for closure when the diagnosis is made in later life because the defect reduces survival in adults who develop progressive pulmonary hypertension. They may also develop atrial tachyarrhythmias, which commonly precipitate heart failure (Table 10.2).

Patients within certain parameters can be selected for transcatheter closure with a septal occluder (Figure 10.12). In those who are unsuitable for the procedure, surgical closure may be considered.

Patent foramen ovale

A patent foramen ovale is a persistent flap-like opening between the atrial septum primum and secundum, which occurs in roughly 25% of adults. With microbubbles injected into a peripheral vein during echocardiography, a patent foramen ovale can be demonstrated by the patient performing and releasing a prolonged Valsalva manoeuvre. Visualisation of microbubbles crossing into the left

Table 10.2 Indications and contraindications for percutaneous closure of atrial septal defects.

Indications

Clinical
- If defect causes symptoms
- Associated cerebrovascular embolic event
- Divers with neurological decompression sickness
- Pulmonary – systemic flow ratio >1.5 and reversible pulmonary hypertension
- Right-to-left atrial shunt and hypoxaemia

Anatomical
- Defects within fossa ovalis (or patent foramen ovale)
- Defects with stretched diameter <38 mm
- Presence of >4-mm rim of tissue surrounding defect

Contraindications
- Sinus venosus defects
- Ostium primum defects
- Ostium secundum defects with other important congenital heart defects requiring surgical correction

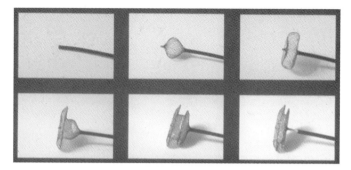

Figure 10.12 Deployment sequence of the Amplatzer septal occluder for closing an atrial septal defect.

atrium reveals a right-to-left shunt mediated by transient reversal of the interatrial pressure gradient.

Although a patent foramen ovale (or an atrial septal aneurysm) has no clinical importance in otherwise healthy adults, it may cause paradoxical embolism in patients with cryptogenic transient ischaemic attack or stroke (up to half of whom have a patent foramen ovale), decompression illness in divers and right-to-left shunting in patients with right ventricular infarction or severe pulmonary hypertension. Patients with patent foramen ovale and paradoxical embolism have an approximate 3.5% yearly risk of recurrent cerebrovascular events.

Secondary preventive strategies are drug treatment (aspirin, clopidogrel or warfarin), surgery or percutaneous closure using a dedicated occluding device (Figure 10.13). The lack of randomised clinical trials directly comparing these options means that optimal treatment remains uncertain. However, percutaneous closure offers a less invasive alternative to traditional surgery and allows patients to avoid potential side effects associated with anticoagulants and interactions with other drugs. In addition, divers taking anticoagulants may experience haemorrhage in the ear, sinus or lung from barotrauma.

Migraine and patent foramen ovale

Studies have indicated that patients with a patent foramen ovale are more likely to suffer from migraine (and vice versa), especially if associated with an aura. In addition, retrospective studies showed that patent foramen ovale closure reduced these migraines,

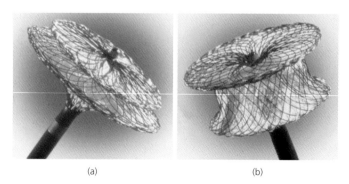

(a)   (b)

Figure 10.13 Amplatzer occluder devices for patent foramen ovale (a) and muscular ventricular septal defects (b).

suggesting that the presence of a shunt may be a trigger. It has been hypothesised that the shunt releases serotonin (a known migraine instigator) from platelets that have been activated by venous bubbles in the left heart. However, the controversial, prospective, randomised MIST study disappointingly failed to show a benefit with closure. At present, there is insufficient evidence to advocate closure for all migraine sufferers with aura.

Congenital ventricular septal defects

Untreated congenital ventricular septal defects that require intervention are rare in adults. Recently, there has been interest in percutaneous device closure of ventricular septal defects acquired as a complication of acute myocardial infarction. However, more experience is necessary to assess the role of this procedure as a primary closure technique or as a bridge to subsequent surgery.

Further reading

Braun MU, Fassbender D, Schoen SP *et al*. Transcatheter closure of patent foramen ovale in patients with cerebral ischaemia. *J Am Coll Cardiol* 2002;**39**:2019–25.

Feldman T, Kar S, Rinaldi M *et al*. Percutaneous mitral repair with the Mitraclip system: safety and midterm durability in the initial EVEREST (Endovascular valve edge-to-edge repair study) cohort. *J Am Coll Cardiol* 2009;**54** (8):686–94.

Inoue K, Lau K-W, Hung J-S. Percutaneous transvenous mitral commissurotomy. In: Grech ED, Ramsdale DR, eds. *Practical Interventional Cardiology*. 2nd ed. London: Martin Dunitz, 2002: 373–87.

Masson JB, Kovac J, Schuler G *et al*. Transcatheter aortic valve implantation: review of the nature, management, and avoidance of procedural complications. *J Am Coll Cardiol Cardiovasc Interv* 2009;**2**(**9**): 811–20.

Nagueh SF, Ommen SR, Lakkis NM *et al*. Comparison of ethanol septal reduction therapy with surgical myectomy for the treatment of hypertrophic obstructive cardiomyopathy *J Am Coll Cardiol* 2001;**38**:1701–6.

Waight DJ, Cao Q-L, Hijazi ZM. Interventional cardiac catheterisation in adults with congenital heart disease. In: Grech ED, Ramsdale DR, eds. *Practical Interventional Cardiology*. 2nd ed. London: Martin Dunitz, 2002:390–406.

Wigle ED, Rakowski H, Kimball BP, Williams WG. Hypertrophic cardiomyopathy: clinical spectrum and treatment. *Circulation* 1995;**92**:1680–92.

Wilkins GT, Weyman AE, Abascal VM, Bloch PC, Palacios IE. Percutaneous balloon dilatation of the mitral valve: an analysis of echocardiographic variables related to outcome and the mechanism of dilatation. *Br Heart J* 1998;**60**:299–308.

CHAPTER 11

New Developments in Percutaneous Coronary Intervention

Julian Gunn[1] and Ever D. Grech[2]

[1]University of Sheffield, Sheffield, UK
[2]South Yorkshire Cardiothoracic Centre, Northern General Hospital, Sheffield, UK

OVERVIEW

- Percutaneous coronary intervention (PCI) can treat most types of coronary artery disease
- Improvements in PCI are dependent upon improvements in technology
- These improvements have been evolutionary as well as revolutionary
- The stent has solved a lot of problems but created others
- The pace of change will continue to accelerate

Introduction

Following on from the 'new device' era of the 1990s, it is commonly stated that there have been three 'quantum leaps' – the balloon, the stent and the drug-eluting stent. However, the dominant developments in recent times have been refinements of the basic tools (Tables 11.1 and 11.2). Hence, the really important advances have been evolutionary, rather than revolutionary. Balloons did not stop evolving in 1980 and similarly, modern stent platforms are infinitely superior to the first hand-crimped, rigid, stainless steel examples (Figure 11.1).

Table 11.1 Interventional devices and their uses.

Device	Use (% of cases)	Types of lesion
Balloon catheter	100	Multiple types
Stent	70–90	Most types
Drug-eluting stent	50–90	High risk of restenosis (possibly all)
Thrombectomy	10–20	Primary angioplasty
Distal protection	3–4	Most vein graft procedures
Stent graft	<1	Aneurysm, arteriovenous malformation, perforation
Cutting devices	1–2	In-stent restenosis, ostial lesions
Rotablator	<1	Calcified, ostial, undilatable lesions
Laser	<1	Occlusions, thrombus, in-stent restenosis
Closure devices	0–100	Femoral access centres use these
Drug-eluting balloons	3–4	In-stent restenosis

ABC of Interventional Cardiology, 2nd edition.
© Ever D. Grech. Published 2011 Blackwell Publishing Ltd.

Table 11.2 Winners and losers in the last 10 years.

Winners	Hanging in there	Losers
Balloons	Bare metal stents	Brachytherapy
Drug-eluting stents	Intracoronary ultrasound	
Thrombectomy	Rotational atherectomy	
Distal protection	Bifurcation stents	
Pressure wires	Lasers	
Radial vascular access	Femoral vascular access	

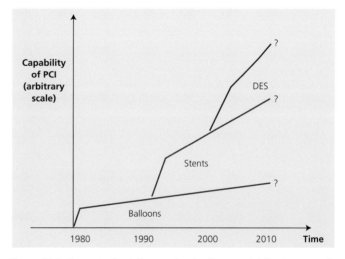

Figure 11.1 Conceptualised diagram showing incremental development of percutaneous coronary intervention (PCI) over the last 30 years. The question marks indicate that even more refinement may be possible in the future. DES, drug-eluting stent.

The changing patient population

In the early days, patients were carefully selected, and the majority were middle-aged, with chronic stable symptoms and proximal, rather simple lesions. The crude equipment available to the interventionist then could only just cope and the technical success rate was quite dismal. Now, the interventionist can be presented with almost any patient, with any pattern of disease, for immediate treatment. The numbers treated are now far greater than before (Table 11.3) and there has been a large increase in the number and proportion of patients with acute coronary syndromes treated by percutaneous coronary intervention (PCI) (Figures 11.2 and 11.3).

Table 11.3 Approximate changes in practice in a 'typical' angioplasty-capable catheter laboratory over the last 20 years.

	Stable angina (Elective)	UA/non-STEMI (Urgent)	STEMI (Emergency)
1990 (%)	80	15	5
2010 (%)	20	40	40

STEMI, ST elevated myocardial infarction; UA, unstable angina.

There remains a substantial number of patients with chronic stable symptoms of ischaemia who require revascularisation. Most isolated lesions in one-, two- and some three-vessel diseases are readily amenable to PCI, and given an informed choice, many patients opt for PCI. Similarly, a proportion of patients have multi-vessel disease with diffuse or adverse features, such as one or more chronic total occlusions (CTOs). Such patients tend to be best treated with bypass surgery. The concept of the multidisciplinary team (MDT) has been developed to discuss many 'grey' cases. In the current era of drug-eluting stents and multi-vessel stenting, the SYNTAX score, a sophisticated lesion-based scoring system reflecting the extent and type of disease, may guide the MDT. High scores indicate superiority for bypass surgery and equivalence for lower scores (Figure 11.4).

There is another, quite large group of patients with significant co-morbidity precluding bypass surgery, but who nevertheless require revascularisation. Advanced age, severe lung disease, a history of stroke, renal disease, anaemia and widespread vascular disease are common reasons for open heart surgery to be avoided. In those circumstances, PCI may offer a reasonable palliation (Figure 11.5).

Chronic total occlusions

In the 1990s, the success rate for PCI recanalisation of a CTO (a vessel that has been completely blocked for more than 3 months) was barely greater than 50%. Since then, great improvements have been made in the technology available to the interventionist. Ranges of guidewires with different properties, notably of tip stiffness, hydrophilicity and penetrating capacity, have been manufactured together with a range of fine probing catheters to provide support as the wire is encouraged to find a microchannel, or even actually bore through the lesion (Figure 11.6). The ultimate combination of

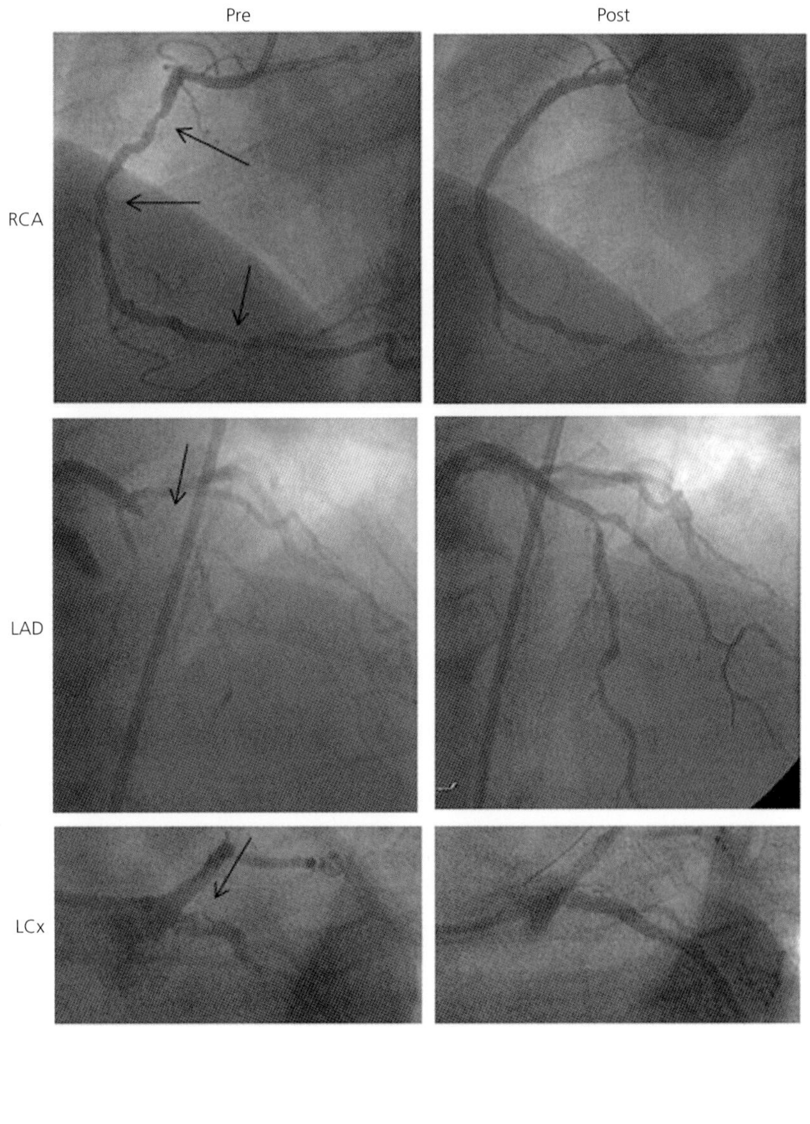

Figure 11.2 A 70-year-old man with acute non-STEMI (non-ST elevated myocardial infarction). Angiography (left three panels) revealed diffuse disease throughout the right coronary artery (RCA), incorporating several particularly tight stenoses, an occlusion of the left anterior descending artery (LAD) and a filling defect in the proximal left circumflex (LCx) artery. The 'culprit' lesion was not obvious. The risk of bypass surgery was very high and PCI was undertaken, with the aim of complete revascularisation. The RCA was stented using conventional techniques. The LAD occlusion was then crossed with a hydrophilic guidewire supported by a probing catheter. A single drug-eluting stent was deployed at the occlusion site, the rest of the diffuse disease being left alone. The LCx filling defect was unchanged throughout, and was also stented. Excellent results were achieved and the patient was discharged the next day.

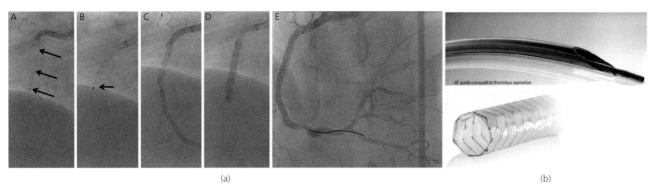

(a)   (b)

Figure 11.3 A 65-year-old man sustained an acute inferior ST elevated myocardial infarction (STEMI). Coronary angiography (a) revealed an occluded dominant right coronary artery (RCA) with a substantial thrombus (A). A coronary guidewire was passed through the occluded segment, and an Export thrombus aspiration catheter (b) was advanced slowly through the thrombus, with application of continuous suction. The marker at the tip of this catheter can be seen over the wire in the middle of the occlusion (B). Flow to the artery was restored but, despite several passes of the aspiration catheter and administration of abciximab via the catheter, there remained a substantial amount of thrombus in the artery (C). An over-and-under pericardium-covered stent graft (c) was then implanted, sealing the thrombus behind its membranous coating (D). The final result was excellent, with restoration of blood flow to the entire artery (E). The patient was discharged 2 days later.

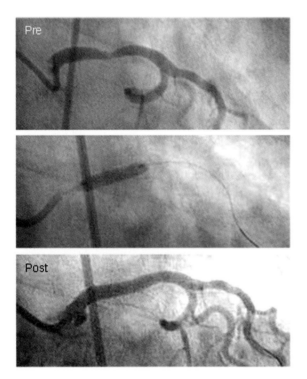

Figure 11.4 A 74-year-old woman with chronic stable angina was found to have a severe single lesion in the body of the left main stem. The SYNTAX score was low, and the patient was offered both percutaneous coronary intervention (PCI) and bypass surgery. After opting for PCI, a single 4-mm stent was successfully deployed at 16 atmospheres pressure. The final result was excellent, and she has had no angina for 4 years.

new techniques and new devices is in 'retrograde' recanalisation of CTOs, whereby a wire is passed from the contralateral coronary artery, through collateral vessels (typically septal branches, from the left anterior descending artery (LAD) to right coronary artery (RCA), or vice versa) to the occlusion, and the lesion may be crossed from distal to proximal. The channel so created can then allow easier passage of an antegrade wire, followed by balloon and

stent. This time-consuming technique requires great patience but may increase the success rate to >80%.

Bifurcation lesions

Bifurcation lesions pose greater technical problems to treat than those within the shaft of a vessel. Adaptations of cylindrical stents to the highly varied geometry and size of bifurcated, stenosed vessels has led to a multitude of techniques. The results of randomised trials indicate that single, rather than double, stent techniques are generally better, leading to the mantra of 'keep it simple'. To address the problem of the bifurcation lesion, stent manufacturers have designed a variety of purpose-made bifurcation stents. Much work remains to be done with these devices, which are limited by bulky profiles, a limited number of sizes and shapes and a lack of drug on their surfaces. Nevertheless, promise is being shown (Figures 11.7 and 11.8).

Diseased vein grafts

Over time, vein grafts themselves become diseased, resulting in stenosis and occlusion. Although the internal mammary artery has a longer lifespan, this too may occlude or stenose. Patients may be elderly, with accrued co-morbidity, and there may be a lack of available conduits. Therefore, repeat bypass surgery – which itself carries a higher risk than the first operation – may not be an attractive option. Frequently, the interventional cardiologist is asked to perform PCI upon diseased bypass grafts or severely diseased and heavily calcified native coronary arteries.

Vein graft PCI requires a different set of skills and technologies. Downstream embolisation of friable debris liberated from the graft, particularly during stent implantation plugs the microvasculature which may cause a 'no-reflow' phenomenon. Protection from this may be provided by positioning a 'basket' or filter distal to the site of stent implantation, allowing capture of any fragments whilst allowing blood flow to continue. A second approach is the use of a

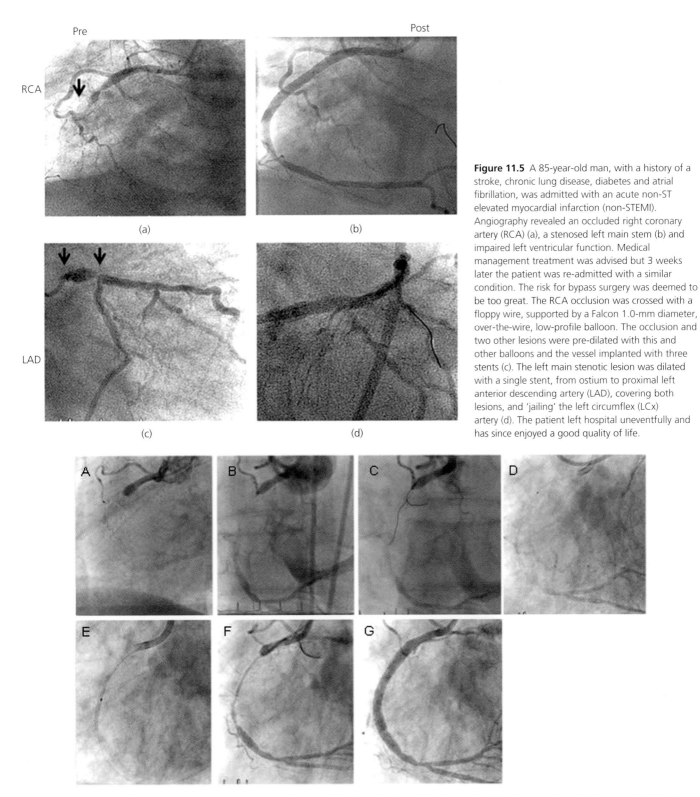

Figure 11.5 A 85-year-old man, with a history of a stroke, chronic lung disease, diabetes and atrial fibrillation, was admitted with an acute non-ST elevated myocardial infarction (non-STEMI). Angiography revealed an occluded right coronary artery (RCA) (a), a stenosed left main stem (b) and impaired left ventricular function. Medical management treatment was advised but 3 weeks later the patient was re-admitted with a similar condition. The risk for bypass surgery was deemed to be too great. The RCA occlusion was crossed with a floppy wire, supported by a Falcon 1.0-mm diameter, over-the-wire, low-profile balloon. The occlusion and two other lesions were pre-dilated with this and other balloons and the vessel implanted with three stents (c). The left main stenotic lesion was dilated with a single stent, from ostium to proximal left anterior descending artery (LAD), covering both lesions, and 'jailing' the left circumflex (LCx) artery (d). The patient left hospital uneventfully and has since enjoyed a good quality of life.

Figure 11.6 A 73-year-old man presented with non-ST elevated myocardial infarction (non-STEMI) 5 months following a previous similar event which had been treated medically. The patient was anaemic and had a shadow on the chest X-ray suspicious for malignancy. A culprit stenosis was found in the left circumflex artery (LCx), together with a chronic total occlusion (CTO) of the right coronary artery (RCA) (A). The LCx was treated with percutaneous coronary intervention (PCI) and the catheter left in the left main stem (LMS). A second arterial sheath was inserted and a catheter was engaged in the RCA. Simultaneous left and right coronary angiography delineated the true extent of the lesion (B). With the support of a 1.5-mm, low-profile, over-the-wire balloon, a stiff guidewire entered a proximal branch repeatedly, and was left there to maintain catheter position. Other guidewires made no headway in the CTO. A third wire advanced through the plaque but followed an eccentric path repeatedly, where it was left (C). With the previous two wires in situ, eventually a Shinobi wire was advanced to the distal end of the plaque, but would not penetrate the distal cap. This wire was exchanged for a crosswire backed up by an NIC 1.1-mm balloon. A final push allowed this wire to enter the vessel lumen distally, its position being confirmed in two projections with contralateral angiography (D). The lesion was then dilated with successive balloons to 2.5 mm at high pressure (E, F), and two long drug-eluting stents of 4.5-mm diameter were implanted. The final result was excellent (G).

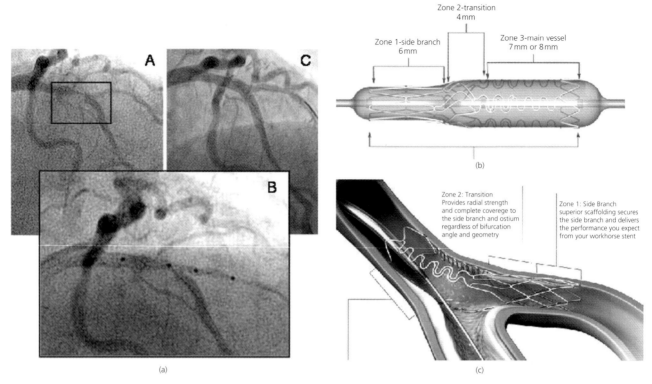

Figure 11.7 A 60-year-old woman who presented with chronic stable angina was referred for percutaneous coronary intervention (PCI) to a lesion (a) in the left anterior descending artery (LAD) immediately proximal to the first diagonal branch (A). A Tryton bifurcation stent (b and c) was deployed. This is a balloon-expandable device with a conventional stent at the tip for the side branch, a funnel-shaped central section to support the ostium of the branch, and a very open rear section (the position of the four markers separating these sections can be seen in B). After pre-dilatation, the device was successfully implanted. The procedure was finished by placing a drug-eluting stent in the LAD across the bifurcation and performing a final kissing balloon dilatation.

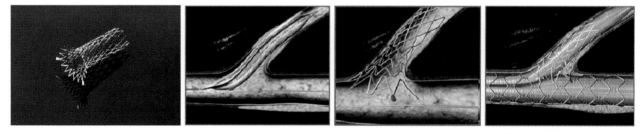

Figure 11.8 Bifurcation procedures are often complicated because of the complex and variable anatomy of the coronary ostia. The nitinol Sideguard stent is an effective option, with a focus on treating the sidebranch of the diseased coronary artery first rather than the main vessel, and allows the preferred stent of choice for the main vessel.

soft, compliant balloon to occlude the graft proximally, causing the blood to stagnate around the lesion. The stent is then deployed and the stagnant blood, together with any debris, is aspirated. A third approach may be to use a 'covered stent', which can contain the friable debris in situ, between the graft wall and mesh (Figure 11.9).

Better imaging

Remarkable developments in digital coronary angiography, which remains the cornerstone of good quality PCI, include 'flat plate' systems, which together with sophisticated software programmes,

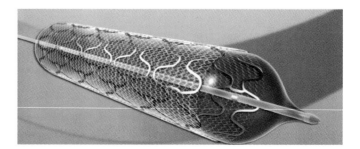

Figure 11.9 An alternative for thrombotic lesions in native vessels or vein grafts is the MGuard polymer mesh-covered stent.

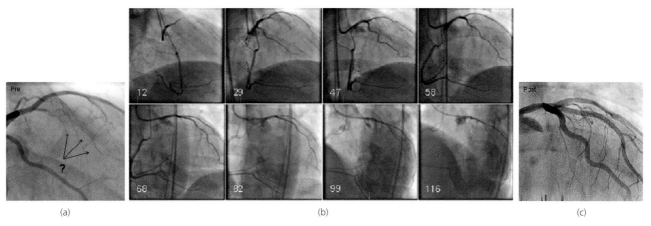

(a) (b) (c)

Figure 11.10 A 42-year-old man with a chronic total occlusion (CTO) of the left anterior descending (LAD) artery. (a) Left coronary angiography in the right anterior oblique projection with cranial angulation failed to reveal the stump, the extent of the lesion or its path. A few wispy antegrade collateral vessels were demonstrated, but a percutaneous coronary intervention (PCI) procedure could not be undertaken on the basis of these images. (b) Rotational angiography with simultaneous contralateral injection of both coronary arteries. The X-ray arm moves through an arc and total of 121 single, two-dimensional images are recorded in a 3-second rotation. A diagnostic right coronary catheter is seen in the right coronary artery (RCA) and a PCI guide catheter in the left coronary artery (LCA). There is a sheath in both groins. The LAD fills from the RCA in the later images (68 onwards; arrows). (c) The lesion was crossed with CTO wires supported by an over-the-wire balloon. After pre-dilatation, the lesion was implanted with a long drug-eluting stent. The final result was excellent.

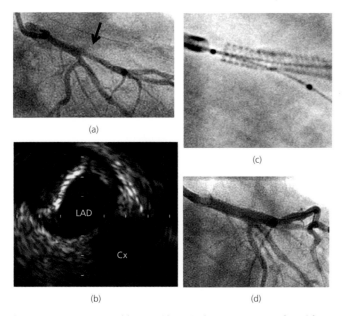

(a)

(b) (c) (d)

Figure 11.11 A 56-year-old man with anginal symptoms was referred for stenting of a proximal left anterior descending artery (LAD) stenosis. It was apparent that the calibre of the LAD at the ostium, proximal to the tightest part of the lesion, was not normal, and the appearance was hazy (a). Intravascular ultrasound (IVUS) was used to determine whether a stent could safely be placed clear of the left main stem. This revealed that the stenosis was severe in proximal LAD and less so at the ostium of the LAD (IVUS images in (b) are shown at the position of the arrow in (a)), with further extension proximally into the left main stem. At the ostium of the LAD, the plaque can be seen to be calcified, eccentric and occupying 50% of the cross-sectional area of the LAD. As stent implantation in the tight part of the lesion would have resulted in plaque disruption at the bifurcation, a large-calibre drug-eluting stent from the left main stem to LAD, covering the entire lesion, was deployed (c). After kissing balloons were deployed, the final result was excellent (d).

provide high image quality, with storage, magnification, subtraction and dose control as standard. However, angiography is a two-dimensional 'luminogram' and provides no information about the vessel wall. It is, however, now possible to perform rotational angiography, in which a single injection of contrast can be combined with a rapid rotation of the X-ray arm in an arc around the patient. This captures a series of >100, single-plane images, each separated by a fraction of a second and about one degree of arc. Rotation may be combined with a software package, which can provide true three-dimensional reconstruction, and give an idea of the orientation of selected coronary arteries and their branches in space, but not fine detail of the lesions (Figure 11.10).

Intravascular ultrasound (IVUS) provides accurate information not only about the lumen but also about the composition of the plaque. It is only required in a small proportion of patients, usually when angiographic images are unclear or uncertain (Figure 11.11). A new intracoronary imaging modality is optical coherence tomography (OCT), which provides extremely high-resolution imaging because it is based on light, rather than sound frequency. Compared with IVUS, OCT images provide much better delineation of vessel layers, leading to clearer visualisation of the vessel plaque, stents and intima. It may also have the potential to identify vulnerable plaques that can cause heart attacks and sudden cardiac death.

Better guidewires

The PCI guidewire is the unsung hero of the PCI procedure. Without a secure guidewire position, no PCI, however innovative, can be undertaken. There is a plethora of guidewires available for PCI nowadays and a typical wire consists of a solid, cylindrical, steel core that tapers towards the tip. Around the tip is usually wound a fine wire, like a coil of spring. This combination, which can be adjusted to produce wires with different shaft and tip stiffnesses, makes the tip flexible and floppy, whilst the proximal shaft is stiff and pushable. Finally, there may be a coating on the wire, usually of a hydrophilic polymer that is lubricious when wet.

The 'workhorse' wire is usually a 'floppy' wire with or without a hydrophilic coating, used for crossing many lesions with minimal risk of trauma. There are some instances when a wire of intermediate stiffness is required. In addition, for a small number of cases, particularly crossing CTOs, wires of increasing stiffness are available. There are also some highly specialised wires, with exceptional stiffness, or a sharp tip, such as the Confianza, which may be used for the retrograde approach in CTOs. Finally, steerable guidewire microcatheters have been designed to negotiate tortuous anatomy, such as hyperacute bends, graft anastomoses and aneurysms.

Better balloons

To meet the many and varied demands, balloon technology is now mature and sophisticated. The principle is simple enough: a shaft to transmit push and transport the dilating fluid; a central

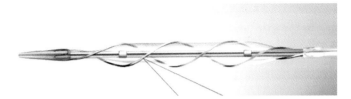

Figure 11.12 The Angiosculpt incising balloon.

wire channel; a balloon envelope, which is wrapped tight with a low profile, has precise non- or semi-compliant characteristics and possesses maximum resistance to puncture; a tip which is low in profile and capable of following a wire through the tightest lesion and a series of joins that are strong but do not spoil the overall profile or performance. Most balloons achieve these targets satisfactorily in over 95% of lesions that require balloon dilatation. The vast majority are of the 'rapid exchange' configuration, rather than the more old-fashioned 'over-the-wire' type.

Most balloons now are made of polymers with semi-compliant characteristics, meaning that a given increase in pressure produces a predictable increment in balloon size. Non-compliant

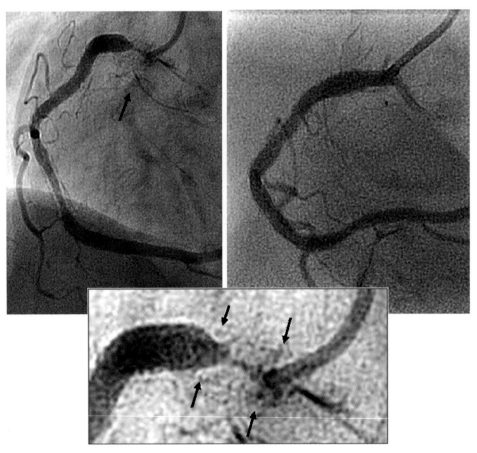

Figure 11.13 A 55-year-old woman underwent stent implantation to the stenosed ostium of her right coronary artery (RCA). This restenosed 3 times, giving rise to recurrent symptoms each time. On the first occasion, simple balloon dilatation was used. On the second, a new drug-eluting stent was deployed inside the first. On the third, the stents were dilated 0.5 mm larger than earlier and a Dior drug-eluting balloon was used to deliver paclitaxel to the site. The fourth and final procedure is shown. On the left panel (and inset) can clearly be seen the (double) stent layers with a large amount of neointima occluding the lumen. On this occasion, a Scoreflex balloon, consisting of a balloon with wires wound around its exterior, was used to both dilate and incise the lesion. Multiple 'cuts' were made, followed by final dilatation with a 5.0 mm non-compliant balloon inflated to 24 atmospheres. The final result was excellent (right panel).

versions, with stiffer polymer, are available to dilate resistant lesions to high pressure without oversizing in adjacent vessel, or for post-dilating stents.

There are some highly specialist balloons. Perhaps, the most important are the very small, low profile ones, used in the recanalisation of CTOs. These sacrifice some of the other qualities of the average balloon for achieving the ultimate crossing profile. The smallest currently available balloon is the NIC Nano with an inflation diameter of just 0.85 mm! It is also useful to keep one or two tiny balloons available in over-the-wire configuration, to allow the exchange of guidewires without losing position.

Super-high pressure balloons are used to treat the otherwise 'undilatable' lesion. The OPN balloon catheter consists of a tough, double membrane balloon, and is almost impervious to bursting by a calcified lesion, and can be safely inflated to >40 atmospheres pressure in an otherwise 'undilatable' lesion. Other balloons come with a frictitious ('knobbly') surface to prevent 'melon-seeding' (Grip), others are supplied with cutting wires on their surface (Angiosculpt) (Figure 11.12) or cutting balloon (now called Flex-Tome), which actually has longitudinal blades on its surface. Some are coated with drugs such as taxol to prevent restenosis (Dior) (Figure 11.13).

Better catheters

There is a wide choice of shape and size of catheters and most operators use a 6F or 7F size catheter, advanced from the femoral, brachial or radial artery. Guide catheters are vital as they allow delivery of balloon or stent smoothly all the way from the outside world to the coronary artery, avoiding damage to the peripheral vessel. In addition, they allow angiographic images, transmit an accurate pressure, prevent stagnant blood clotting on its surface and provide extra push or backup when required without trauma to the vessel.

Small calibre catheters are useful for radial procedures in straightforward lesions, and can even be advanced right down a coronary artery to deliver a stent to a lesion. Large calibre catheters are useful for complex procedures, requiring special equipment (such as large rotablator burrs), bifurcation work employing bulky bifurcation stents or the simultaneous deployment of two stents (Figure 11.14), whilst maintaining contrast injection and accurate pressure measurement and avoiding friction between stents and other devices.

Better stent platforms

The transformation from the very first human stent implants to the current range of drug-eluting stents has been dramatic. The first simple, slotted tube, stainless steel devices that were hand crimped onto a balloon, was followed by pre-mounted stents with a much improved profile. Stent geometry was made more sophisticated, so that the undeployed stent/balloon was more trackable, and the vessel coverage more even. Stents with thin struts were shown to be less prone to restenosis than those with thick ones; and other alloys were used, such as cobalt, chromium or platinum, which had similar radial strength to stainless steel despite thinner struts. At the

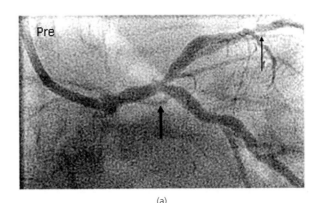

(a)

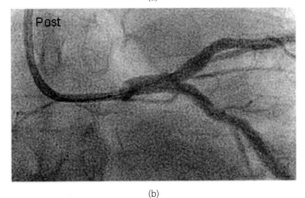

(b)

Figure 11.14 (a) A 68-year-old woman with chronic stable angina, a bifurcation stenosis of the left main stem (left arrow) and a lesion in the proximal left anterior descending artery (LAD) (right arrow). She had severe peripheral vascular disease, with absent femoral pulses and significant carotid artery disease. Cardiac surgery was thought to be excessively hazardous. As percutaneous coronary intervention (PCI), performed from an arm artery, would involve a simultaneous kissing stent technique for the left main stem lesion, a large-calibre catheter was needed. Therefore, a 7.5F sheathless Eaucath (external diameter the same as that of a 6F sheath) was deployed from the right radial artery and the procedure was successful (b).

same time, improved deployment methods (notably high-pressure post-dilatation) allow harsh anticoagulation regimens to be all but eliminated. Patients are now prescribed two different antiplatelet agents, with attendant reduction in bleeding complications.

The impact of drug-eluting stents in reducing restenosis has been considerable. A concern has been the potential for these devices to be associated with delayed healing and a low risk of late stent thrombosis, which may be devastating. A new generation of drug-eluting stents has emerged, with even lower restenosis rates and virtual elimination of late stent thrombosis.

Better adjunct therapy

In the early days of balloon angioplasty, the critical importance of the circulating platelet was under-appreciated. The cyclooxygenase inhibitor aspirin has been a constant adjunct therapy for PCI, and is effective. Stent implantation requires more complete platelet inhibition and the thienopyridine clopidogrel fulfils that function. However, clopidogrel resistance has been a source of concern, but the newer replacements (prasugrel and ticagrelor) surmount this problem. Intravenous glycoprotein IIb/IIIa inhibitors such as abciximab also have a place in PCI especially during the treatment of some acute coronary syndromes. The anti-thrombin agent heparin is still used in the vast majority of PCI procedures. Seeking to replace heparin and abciximab are the direct thrombin inhibitors, such as bivalirudin. However, it is an expensive drug.

In supporting the arterial circulation in patients with cardiogenic shock, the most widely used physical adjunct to PCI is the intra-aortic balloon pump. Its use is less clear in high-risk PCI cases, especially when left ventricular function is particularly poor, or when there is acute vessel closure. Other left ventricular assist devices are available, and one of the most promising is the Impella, an axial flow pump that sucks blood out of the left ventricle and deposits it in the aorta.

Further reading

Erbel R, Di Mario C, Bartunek J et al. Temporary scaffolding of coronary arteries with bioabsorbable magnesium stents: a prospective, non-randomised multicentre trial. *Lancet* 2007;**369**:1869–75.

Lagerqvist B, James SK, Stenestrand U, Lindbäck J, Nilsson T, Wallentin L; SCAAR Study Group. Long term outcomes with drug eluting stents versus bare metal stents in Sweden. *New Engl J Med* 2007;**356**:1009–19.

Lee YP, Tay E, Lee CH et al. Endothelial progenitor cell capture stent implantation in patients with ST-segment elevation myocardial infarction: one year follow-up. *EuroIntervention* 2010;**5**:698–702.

Moses JW, Leon MB, Popma JJ et al. Sirolimus eluting stents versus standard stents in patients with stenosis in a native coronary artery. *New Engl J Med* 2003;**349**:1315–23.

Weintraub WS, Spertus JA, Kolm P et al. Effect of PCI on quality of life in patients with stable coronary disease. *New Engl J Med* 2008;**359**:677–87.

CHAPTER 12

Percutaneous Interventional Electrophysiology

Gerald C. Kaye

Princess Alexandra Hospital, Woolloongabba, Brisbane, QLD, Australia

---

OVERVIEW

- Most types of supraventricular tachycardia (SVT) are curable with ablation
- Atrial flutter can be cured with ablation with a low complication rate and should be considered first-line treatment
- Patients with ventricular pre-excitation (the Wolff–Parkinson–White syndrome) need cardiological referral
- Patients with structural heart disease and recurrent syncope/presyncope need urgent cardiological assessment
- Patients with recurrent palpitations and structural heart disease need cardiology referral

---

Prior to the 1980s, cardiac electrophysiology was primarily used to confirm mechanisms of arrhythmia, with management mainly by pharmacological means. However, recognised shortcomings in antiarrhythmic drugs spurred the development of non-pharmacological treatments, particularly radiofrequency ablation.

The two major mechanisms by which arrhythmias (Figure 12.1) occur are automaticity and re-entrant excitation (Table 12.1). Most

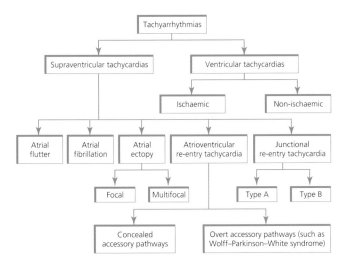

Figure 12.1 Classification of arrhythmias.

ABC of Interventional Cardiology, 2nd edition.
© Ever D. Grech. Published 2011 Blackwell Publishing Ltd.

Table 12.1 Mechanisms and classification of arrhythmias.

Unicellular
- Enhanced automaticity
- Triggered activity – early or delayed after depolarisations

Multicellular
- Re-entry
- Electrotonic interaction
- Mechanico-electrical coupling

Table 12.2 Arrhythmias associated with re-entry.

- Sinus node re-entry tachycardia
- Junctional re-entry tachycardia (atrioventricular nodal re-entrant tachycardia – AVNRT)
- Atrioventricular reciprocating tachycardias (AVRT – such as Wolf–Parkinson–White syndrome)
- Atrial flutter
- Atrial fibrillation
- Ventricular tachycardia

arrhythmias are of the re-entrant type and require two or more pathways that are anatomically or functionally distinct but in electrical contact (Table 12.2). The conduction in one pathway must also be slowed to a sufficient degree to allow recovery of the other, so that an electrical impulse may then re-enter the area of slowed conduction (Figure 12.2).

Intracardiac electrophysiological studies

Intracardiac electrophysiological studies give valuable information about normal and abnormal electrophysiology of intracardiac structures. They are used to confirm the mechanism of an arrhythmia, to delineate its anatomical substrate and to ablate it. The electrical stability of the ventricles can also be assessed, as can the effects of an antiarrhythmic regimen (Table 12.3).

Atrioventricular conduction

Electrodes positioned at various sites in the heart give only limited data about intracardiac conduction during sinus rhythm at rest.

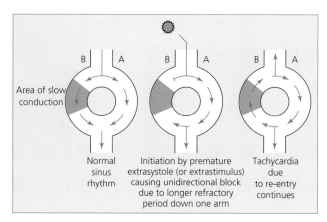

Figure 12.2 Mechanism of a re-entry circuit. An excitation wave is propagated at a normal rate down path A, but slowly down path B. An excitation wave from an extrasystole now encounters the slow pathway (B), which is still refractory, creating unidirectional block. There is now retrograde conduction from path A, which coincides with the end of the refractory period in path B. This gives rise to a persistent circus movement.

Table 12.3 Indications for electrophysiological studies.

Investigation of symptoms
- History of persistent palpitations
- Recurrent syncope
- Presyncope with impaired left ventricular function

Interventions
- Radiofrequency ablation – accessory pathways, junctional tachycardias, atrial flutter, atrial fibrillation
- Investigation of documented arrhythmias (narrow and broad complex) with or without radiofrequency ablation
- Assessment or ablation of ventricular arrhythmias

Contraindications
- Acute myocardial infarction, severe aortic stenosis, unstable coronary disease, left main stem stenosis, substantial electrolyte disturbance

'Stressing' the system allows more information to be generated, particularly concerning atrioventricular nodal conduction and the presence of accessory pathways (Figure 12.3).

By convention, the atria are paced at 100 beats/minute for eight beats. The ninth beat is premature (extrastimulus), and the AH interval (the time between the atrial signal (A) and the His signal (H), which represents atrioventricular node conduction time) is measured. This sequence is repeated with the ninth beat made increasingly premature. In normal atrioventricular nodal conduction, the AH interval gradually increases as the extrastimulus becomes more premature and is graphically represented as the atrioventricular nodal curve (Figure 12.4). The gradual prolongation of the AH interval (decremental conduction) is a feature that rarely occurs in accessory pathway conduction.

Retrograde ventriculoatrial conduction

Retrograde conduction through the atrioventricular node is assessed by pacing the ventricle and observing conduction back into the atria. The coronary sinus electrode is critically important

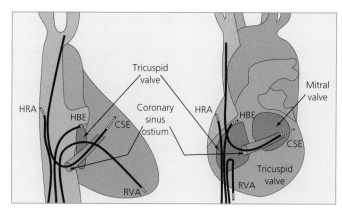

Figure 12.3 Diagrams showing position of pacing or recording electrodes in the heart in the right anterior oblique and left anterior oblique views (views from the right and left sides of the chest respectively). HRA, high right atrial electrode, usually on the lateral wall or appendage; HBE, His bundle electrode, on the medial aspect of the tricuspid valve; RVA, right ventricular apex; CSE, coronary sinus electrode, which records electrical deflections from the left side of the heart between the atrium and ventricle.

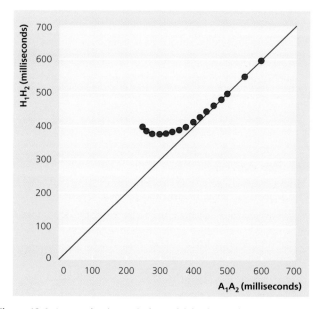

Figure 12.4 A normal atrioventricular nodal 'hockey stick' curve during antegrade conduction of atrial extrastimuli. As the atrial extrastimulus (A_1–A_2) becomes more premature, the AH interval (H_1–H_2) shortens until the atrioventricular node becomes functionally refractory.

for this. It lies between the left ventricle and atrium and provides information about signals passing over the left side of the heart. The sequence of signals that pass from the ventricle to the atria is called the *retrograde activation sequence*. Retrograde conduction is not present in everybody.

If an accessory pathway is present, this sequence changes: with left-sided pathways, there is an apparent 'short circuit' in the coronary sinus with a shorter ventriculoatrial conduction time. This is termed a *concealed pathway*, as its effect cannot be seen on a surface electrocardiogram. It conducts retrogradely only, unlike in Wolff–Parkinson–White syndrome, where the pathway is bidirectional (Figure 12.5). Often, intracardiac electrophysiological

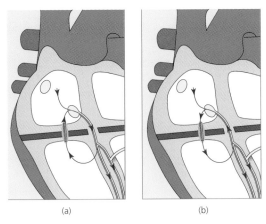

Figure 12.5 Mechanisms for orthodromic (a) and antedromic (b) atrioventricular re-entrant tachycardia.

studies are the only way to confirm concealed accessory pathways, which form the basis for many tachycardias with narrow QRS complexes (Figure 12.6).

Supraventricular tachycardia

Supraventricular tachycardias have narrow QRS complexes with rates usually between 150 and 250 beats/minute. The two common mechanisms involve re-entry due to either an accessory pathway (overt as in Wolf–Parkinson–White syndrome or concealed) or junctional re-entry tachycardia.

Accessory pathways

These lie between the atria and ventricles in the atrioventricular ring, and most are left sided. Arrhythmias are usually initiated by an extrasystole or, during intracardiac electrophysiological studies, by an extrastimulus, either atrial or ventricular. The extrasystole produces delay within the atrioventricular node, allowing the signal which has passed to the ventricle to re-enter the atria via the accessory pathway. This may reach the atrioventricular node before the next sinus beat arrives but when the atrioventricular node is no longer refractory, thus allowing the impulse to pass down the His bundle and back up to the atrium through the pathway. As ventricular depolarisation is normal, QRS complexes are narrow. This circuit accounts for over 90% of supraventricular tachycardias in Wolf–Parkinson–White syndrome. Rarely, the circuit is reversed, and the QRS complexes are broad as the ventricles are fully pre-excited. This rhythm is often misdiagnosed as ventricular in origin.

Treatment

Pathway ablation effects a complete cure by destroying the arrhythmia substrate. Steerable ablation catheters allow most areas within the heart to be reached. The left atrium can be accessed either retrogradely via the aortic valve, by flexing the catheter tip through the mitral valve, or transseptally across the atrial septum. Radiofrequency energy is delivered to the atrial insertion of a pathway and usually results in either a rapid disappearance of pre-excitation on

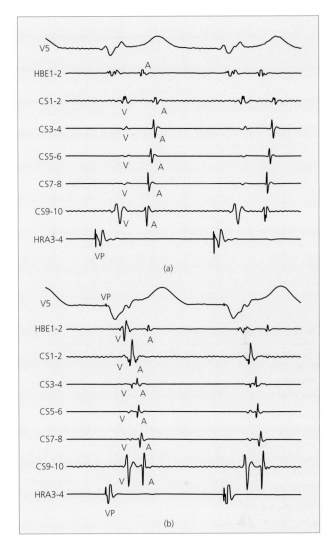

Figure 12.6 Coronary sinus electrode signals, with poles CS9–10 placed proximally near the origin of the coronary sinus and poles 1–2 placed distally reflecting changes in the left ventricular–left atrial free wall. (a) Normal retrograde activation sequence with depolarisation passing from the ventricle back through the atrioventricular node to the right atrium and simultaneously across the coronary sinus to the left atrium. (b) Retrograde activation sequence in the presence of an accessory pathway in the free wall of the left ventricle showing a shorter ventriculoatrial (VA) time than would be expected in the distal coronary sinus electrodes (CS1–2). Such a pathway would not be discernible from a surface electrocardiogram.

the surface electrocardiogram or, in the case of concealed pathways, normalisation of the retrograde activation sequence (Figure 12.7). Accessory pathway ablation is 95% successful. Failure occurs from an inability to accurately map pathways or difficulty in delivering enough energy, usually because of positional instability of the catheter. Complications are rare (<0.5%) and are related to vascular access – femoral artery aneurysms or, with left-sided pathways, embolic cerebrovascular accidents.

Junctional re-entry tachycardia

This is the commonest cause of paroxysmal supraventricular tachycardia. The atrioventricular nodal curve shows a sudden

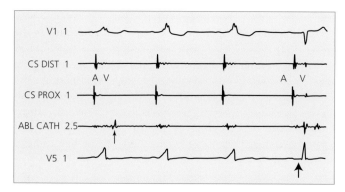

Figure 12.7 Surface electrocardiogram leads V1 and V5 and signals from the distal coronary sinus electrodes (CS dist), proximal electrodes (CS prox) and the tip of the ablation catheter (ABL CAT I) during pathway ablation to treat Wolff–Parkinson–White syndrome. The onset of radiofrequency energy (thin arrow) produces loss of pre-excitation after two beats with a narrow complex QRS seen at the fourth beat (broad arrow). Prolongation of the AV signal in the coronary sinus occurs when pre-excitation is lost.

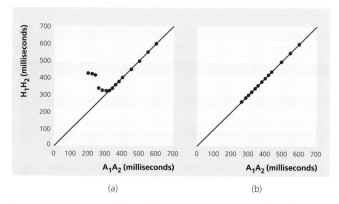

Figure 12.8 Atrioventricular nodal curves. In a patient with slow–fast junctional re-entrant tachycardia (a), there is a 'jump' in atrioventricular nodal conduction when conduction changes from the fast to the slow pathway. In a patient with accessory pathways conducting antegradely (such as Wolff–Parkinson–White syndrome), there is no slowing of conduction as seen in the normal atrioventricular node, and the curve reflects conduction exclusively over the pathway (b).

unexpected prolongation of the AH interval known as a *jump* in the interval (Figure 12.8). The tachycardia is initiated at or shortly after the jump. The jump occurs because of the presence of two pathways – one slowly conducting but with relatively rapid recovery (the slow pathway), the other rapidly conducting but with relatively slow recovery (the fast pathway), called *duality of atrioventricular nodal conduction*. This disparity between conduction speed and recovery allows re-entrance to occur. On a surface electrocardiogram, the QRS complexes are narrow, and the P waves are often absent or distort the terminal portion of the QRS complex. These arrhythmias can often be terminated by critically timed atrial or ventricular extrastimuli.

In the common type of junctional re-entry tachycardia (type A) the circuit comprises antegrade depolarisation of the slow pathway and retrograde depolarisation of the fast pathway. Rarely (<5% of junctional re-entry tachycardias), the circuit is reversed (type B). The slow and fast pathways are anatomically separate,

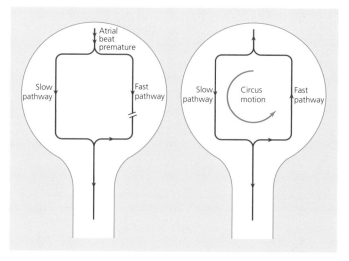

Figure 12.9 Mechanism of slow–fast junctional re-entrant tachycardia. A premature atrial impulse finds the fast pathway refractory, allowing retrograde conduction back up to the atria.

with both inputting to an area called the *compact atrioventricular node* (Figure 12.9). The arrhythmia can be cured by mapping and ablating either the slow or fast pathway, and overall success occurs in 98% of cases. Irreversible complete heart block requiring a permanent pacemaker occurs in 1–2% of cases, with the risk being higher for fast pathway ablation. Therefore, slow pathway ablation is the more usual approach.

Atrial flutter

Atrial flutter is a macro re-entrant circuit within the right atrium. There are two common types: typical and atypical. The critical area of slow conduction lies at the base of the right atrium in the region of the slow atrioventricular nodal pathway. Producing a discrete linear line of ablation between the tricuspid annulus and the inferior vena cava gives a line of electrical block and is associated with a high success rate in terminating flutter. Flutter responds poorly to standard antiarrhythmic drugs, and ablation carries a sufficiently impressive success rate to make it a standard treatment.

Atrial fibrillation (AF)

Although atrial fibrillation (AF) used to be thought of as a non-curable chaotic rhythm, its management has changed dramatically in recent years. There are three clinically recognised types of atrial fibrillation: paroxysmal, persistent and chronic. In paroxysmal AF, there are foci of atrial ectopy arising within the pulmonary veins at their junction with the left atrium (Figure 12.10). These foci fire repetitively, giving rise to frequent ectopy within the atria (Figure 12.11). Over time, it is believed that the frequency increases to a degree where the rhythm breaks down into multiple small re-entrant wavelets giving rise to persistent or chronic AF. Initial studies using radiofrequency ablation showed that by ablating these foci within the veins, the frequency of AF was significantly reduced. A serious complication of ablating within the veins is pulmonary

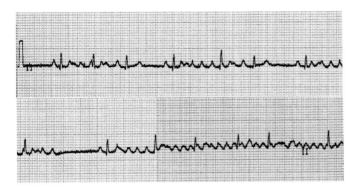

Figure 12.10 Electrocardiogram (ECG) rhythm strip showing sinus rhythm with increasingly frequent atrial ectopy culminating in a paroxysm of atrial fibrillation (lower ECG). The ectopy is referred to as *focal firing* as the atrial ectopics arise from the pulmonary veins (see text). Another term for atrial fibrillation of this nature is *focal AF*.

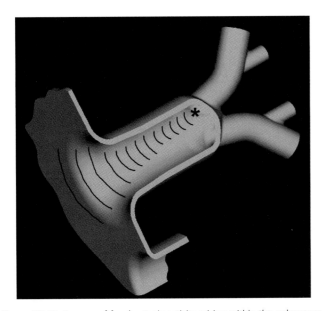

Figure 12.11 An area of focal ectopic activity arising within the pulmonary vein and depolarising atrial tissue. There are often many of these ectopics within each vein and all require isolation to effect a cure for atrial fibrillation (AF).

vein stenosis. This can be avoided by ablating outside the veins as they enter the atria, a technique known as *pulmonary vein isolation*. Although the foci still fire repetitively, the impulse no longer spreads to the atria. Some centres now claim that paroxysmal AF can be cured with this approach, although the long-term effectiveness over many years is still unclear. Persistent and chronic AF are also amenable to this approach but the results are less impressive and the procedure is currently long and complex. In addition to pulmonary vein isolation, extensive ablation is also required within the body of the left atrium. However, by combining computed tomography (CT)-guided imaging of the left atrium with the electrophysiological signals, the safety and efficacy of ablation has been steadily improving and it is now being used as a standard approach for the treatment of symptomatic patients with AF in whom therapy with two or more drugs has failed.

AF can also be treated surgically with a high success rate with a procedure known as the *Maze operation* (first performed in the 1980s). Electrical dissociation of the atria from the great veins was carried out by surgical excision of the pulmonary and vena caval veins from their insertion sites and then suturing them back. The scarred areas acted as insulation, preventing atrial wavefronts from circulating within the atria. This procedure is carried out during other forms of cardiac surgery in patients with previous AF and is rarely recommended as a primary therapy now that catheter ablation has become widespread.

Ventricular tachycardia

Ventricular tachycardia carries a serious adverse prognosis, particularly in the presence of coronary artery disease and impaired ventricular function. Treatment options include drugs, surgical intervention (bypass or infrequently now, arrhythmia surgery) and implantable defibrillators, either alone or in combination. Ventricular tachycardia can be broadly divided into two groups – ischaemic and non-ischaemic. The latter includes arrhythmias arising from the right ventricular outflow tract and those associated with cardiomyopathies.

Since the radiofrequency energy of an ablation catheter is destructive only at the site of the catheter tip, this approach lends itself more to arrhythmias where a discrete abnormality can be described, such as non-ischaemic ventricular tachycardia. In ischaemic ventricular tachycardia, where the abnormal substrate often occurs over a wide area, the success rate is lower.

Ideally, the arrhythmia should be haemodynamically stable, reliably initiated with ventricular pacing and mapped to a localised area within the ventricle. In many cases, however, this is not possible. The arrhythmia may be unstable after initiation, making mapping difficult. The circuit may also lie deep within the ventricular wall and cannot be fully ablated. However, detailed intracardiac maps can be made with multipolar catheters (Figure 12.12). Newer

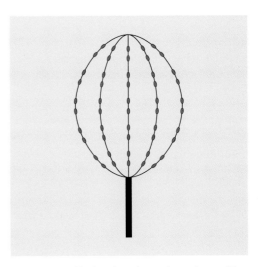

Figure 12.12 Diagram of basket-shaped mapping catheter with several recording electrodes (red dots). The basket retracts into a catheter for placement in either the atria or ventricles. Once it is in position, retraction of the catheter allows the basket to expand.

approaches include the use of a non-contact mapping catheter, which floats freely within the ventricles but senses myocardial electrical circuits, or electroanatomical systems that integrate CT- or magnetic resonance imaging (MRI)-guided images with electrical signals onto a single computer screen.

Although the overall, long-term success rate for radiofrequency ablation of ischaemic ventricular tachycardia is only about 65%, this will increase as technology improves.

Current energy sources

The commonest source of energy used is radiofrequency and for many cases, for example, for accessory pathways and slow pathway ablation, it is highly effective. Increasingly, a deeper lesion needs to be given for conditions such as for atrial flutter, ventricular tachycardia and pulmonary vein isolation for AF. To achieve a deeper burn without producing significant eschar, irrigation-tipped catheters have been developed. These have small irrigation ports at the tip through which saline at room temperature is pumped. This cools the catheter tip as the energy is given and allows more energy to be delivered, producing a deeper burn. It is used extensively for ventricular tachycardias, pulmonary vein isolation and, in some cases, for atrial flutter.

Cryoablation

This involves tissue lysis and death by freezing using liquid nitrogen pumped to the tip of the catheter. The advantage is that tissues can be cooled initially before a full destructive lesion is applied. If there are any issues with cooling, for example, complete heart block during slow pathway ablation, then the tissues can be warmed up and conduction restored. Cryoablation is safer around the AV nodal area and is used particularly in children. The relapse rate, however, is higher than with radiofrequency. Cryoablation for AF using a balloon inserted into the origin of the pulmonary vein is an increasingly popular technique and is proving as effective as radiofrequency.

Newer catheters

New catheter design is changing the way energy is delivered. A 'branding iron' technique using multipolar catheters applied at the ostium of the pulmonary veins is increasingly being used for AF ablation. This allows radiofrequency energy to be cycled between the various poles, producing a circumferential lesion.

Conclusion

The electrophysiological approach to treating arrhythmias has been revolutionised by radiofrequency ablation. Better computerised mapping, improved catheters and more efficient energy delivery have enabled many arrhythmias to be treated and cured. The ability to ablate some forms of atrial fibrillation and improvement in ablation of ventricular tachycardia is heralding a new age of electrophysiology. Ten years ago it could have been said that electrophysiologists were a relatively benign breed of cardiologists who did little harm but little good either. That has emphatically changed, and it can now be attested that electrophysiologists exact the only true cure in cardiology.

Further reading

Calkins H, Leon AR, Deam AG, Kalbfleisch SJ, Langberg JJ, Morady F. Catheter ablation of atrial flutter using radiofrequency energy. *Am J Cardiol* 1994;**73**:353–6.

Earley MJ, Schilling RJ. Catheter and surgical ablation of atrial fibrillation. *Heart* 2006;**92**;266–74.

Jackman WM, Beckman KJ, McClelland JH *et al.* Treatment of supraventricular tachycardia due to atrioventricular nodal re-entry by radiofrequency catheter ablation of the slow-pathway conduction. *N Engl J Med* 1992;**327**:313–18.

McGuire MA, Janse MJ. New insights on the anatomical location of components of the reentrant circuit and ablation therapy for atrioventricular reentrant tachycardia. *Curr Opin Cardiol* 1995;**10**:3–8.

Olgin JE, Zipes DE. Specific arrhythmias: diagnosis and treatment. In: Braunwald E, Zipes DP, Libby P, eds. *Heart Disease*. 6th ed. Philadelphia: Saunders, 2001:1877–85.

Schilling RJ, Peter NS, Davies DW Feasibility of a non-contact catheter for endocardial mapping of human ventricular tachycardia. *Circulation* 1999;**99**:2543–52.

CHAPTER 13

Implantable Devices for Treating Tachyarrhythmias

Gerald C. Kaye

Princess Alexandra Hospital, Woolloongabba, Brisbane, QLD, Australia

---

OVERVIEW

- Patients surviving a cardiac arrest not due to a reversible cause require assessment for a defibrillator
- Poor left ventricular (LV) function (ejection fraction of <30%) predicts an increased risk of sudden cardiac death (SCD).
- Empirical amiodarone therapy is ineffective for prevention of SCD
- Implantable cardioverter defibrillators (ICDs) are effective at preventing sudden death in patients with poor LV function
- ICDs are effective at preventing cardiac death in patients presenting with life-threatening ventricular arrhythmias

---

Pacing treatment for tachycardia control has achieved success, in both supraventricular and ventricular tachycardia. Pacing termination for ventricular tachycardia has been more challenging, but an understanding of arrhythmia mechanisms, combined with increasingly sophisticated pacemakers and the ability to deliver intracardiac pacing and shocks, have led to success with implantable cardioverter defibrillators (ICDs).

Mechanisms of pacing termination for ventricular tachycardias

Overdrive pacing

This is the standard approach for terminating both supraventricular and ventricular tachycardias. It is painless, quick, highly effective and associated with low battery drain of the pacemaker. Implantation of devices for terminating supraventricular tachycardias is now obsolete because of the high success rate of ablation procedures. Overdrive pacing for ventricular tachycardia is often successful but may cause acceleration or induce ventricular fibrillation. Therefore, any device capable of pace termination of ventricular tachycardia must also have defibrillatory capability.

Implantable cardioverter defibrillators (ICDs)

The first implantable defibrillator was implanted in 1980. The early operations involved a sternotomy or sometimes a thoracotomy

associated with 3–5% mortality. The defibrillation electrodes were patches sewn onto the myocardium, and leads were tunnelled subcutaneously to the device, which was implanted in an abdominal rectus sheath pocket. Early devices were large and often shocked patients inappropriately, mainly because these relatively unsophisticated units could not distinguish ventricular tachycardia from supraventricular tachycardia. Current systems are much smaller, have transvenous leads and the generator is implanted subcutaneously (Figure 13.1).

Current implantation procedures

Modern ICDs are transvenous systems, no thoracotomy is required and implantation mortality is about 0.5%. The device is implanted either subcutaneously, as for a pacemaker, in the left or right deltopectoral area, or, if necessary, subpectorally in thin patients to prevent the device eroding the skin.

The ventricular lead tip is positioned in the right ventricle, usually the apex (the outflow tract can be used if necessary), and a second lead can be positioned in the right atrial appendage for dual-chamber pacing if required (Figure 13.2). This provides sensing of the atrium allowing better discrimination between atrial and ventricular tachycardias. The ventricular defibrillator lead has either one or two shocking coils. For two-coil leads, one is proximal (usually within the superior vena cava) and one is distal (right ventricle) (Figure 13.3). During implantation, the unit is tested under conscious sedation. This is to establish satisfactory sensing between sinus rhythm and ventricular fibrillation as well as pacing and defibrillation thresholds. Defibrillatory thresholds should be at least 10 joules less than the maximum output of the defibrillator (30–35 joules).

All modern defibrillators have the ability to record intracardiac electrograms (Figure 13.4). This allows more accurate diagnosis of each arrhythmia episode and can determine whether anti-tachycardia pacing or defibrillation was appropriate. If treatment has been inappropriate, then programming changes can be made with a programming unit placed over the defibrillator site.

Current devices use anti-tachycardia pacing combined with low- and high-energy shocks (Figure 13.5)– known as *tiered therapy*. Anti-tachycardia pacing is a valuable treatment modality and is often successful at tachycardia termination. Most ventricular arrhythmias are re-entrant. The pacing train penetrates the

---

ABC of Interventional Cardiology, 2nd edition.

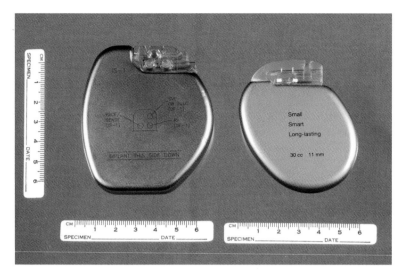

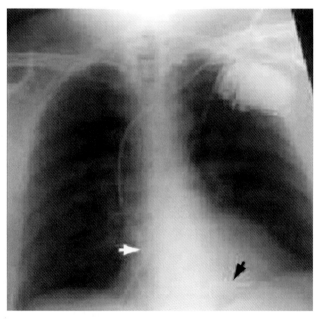

Figure 13.1 The size and volume of implantable cardioverter defibrillators (ICDs) have significantly reduced over the years. The device on the left is only 3 years older than the one on the right, which is much smaller and more compact. Apart from the marked reduction in size, the implant technique and the required hardware have also dramatically improved – from the sternotomy approach with four leads and abdominal implantation to the present two-lead transvenous endocardial approach that is no more invasive than a pacemaker implant.

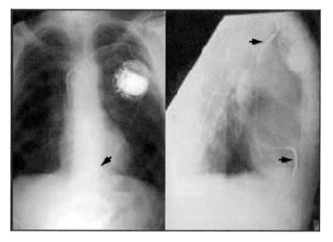

Figure 13.3 Posteroanterior and lateral chest radiographs of transvenous implantable cardioverter defibrillator showing the proximal and distal lead coils (arrows).

Figure 13.2 Chest radiograph of a dual-chamber implantable cardioverter defibrillator with a dual coil ventricular lead (black arrow) and right atrial lead (white arrow).

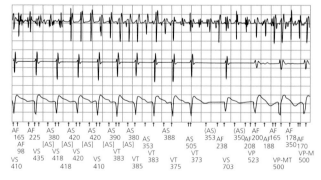

Figure 13.4 Intracardiac electrograms from an implantable cardioverter defibrillator. Upper recording is an intra-atrial electrogram, which shows atrial fibrillation. Middle and lower tracings are intracardiac electrograms rom the ventricle.

arrhythmia circuit and produces an area of refractoriness ahead of the circulating wavefront, thereby terminating the arrhythmia. Anti-tachycardia pacing is painless and can take the form of adaptive burst pacing, with cycle length usually about 80–90% of that of the ventricular tachycardia. Pacing bursts can be fixed (constant cycle length) or autodecremental, when the pacing burst accelerates (each cycle length becomes shorter as the pacing train progresses). Should anti-tachycardia pacing fail, low-energy shocks are given first to try to terminate ventricular tachycardia with the minimum of pain (as some patients remain conscious despite rapid ventricular tachycardia) and reduce battery drain, thereby increasing device longevity.

With the advent of dual-chamber systems and improved diagnostic algorithms, shocking is mostly avoided during supraventricular tachycardia. Even in single-lead systems, there are algorithms which

allow differentiation of some types of supraventricular tachycardia, particularly atrial fibrillation and ventricular tachycardia. There is a rate stability function, which assesses cycle length variability and helps to exclude atrial fibrillation. However, inappropriate shocks still remain a problem for both single-lead and dual chamber

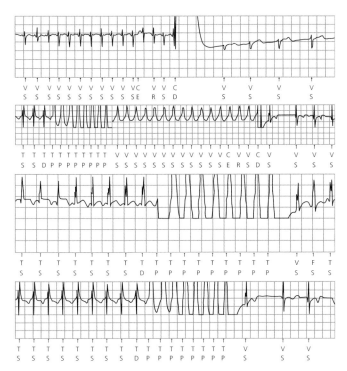

Figure 13.5 Intracardiac electrogram from implantable cardioverter defibrillators. Top: Ventricular tachycardia terminated with a single high-energy shock. Second down: Ventricular tachycardia acceleration after unsuccessful ramp pacing, which was then terminated with a shock. Third down: Unsuccessful fixed burst pacing. Bottom: Successful ramp pacing termination of ventricular tachycardia.

ICDs although the latter provide the best means of detecting atrial arrhythmias.

Device recognition of tachyarrhythmias is based mainly on the tachycardia cycle length, which can initiate anti-tachycardia pacing or low-energy or high-energy shocks. With rapid tachycardias, the device can be programmed to give a shock as first-line treatment.

Complications

These include infection; perforation, displacement, fracture or insulation breakdown of the leads; oversensing or undersensing of the arrhythmia and inappropriate shocks for sinus tachycardia or supraventricular tachycardia. Psychological problems are common, and counselling plays an important role. Regular follow-up is required. If antiarrhythmic drugs are taken concurrently, the potential use of an ICD is reduced.

Precautions – after patient death, the device must be switched off before removal, otherwise a severe electric shock can be delivered to the person removing the device. The implanting centre or local hospital should be informed that the patient has died and arrangements can usually be made to turn the ICD off. The device *must* be removed before cremation.

Driving and implantable cardioverter defibrillators

The UK Driver and Vehicle Licensing Agency recommends that group 1 (private motor car) licence holders are prohibited from driving for 6 months after implantation of a defibrillator when there have been preceding symptoms of an arrhythmia. If an appropriate shock is delivered within this period, driving is withheld for a further 6 months.

Any change in device programming or antiarrhythmic drugs means a month of abstinence from driving, and all patients must remain under regular review. There is a 5-year prohibition on driving if treatment or the arrhythmia is associated with incapacity.

If the device has been implanted prophylactically (primary prevention), driving is withheld for a month.

Drivers holding a group 2 licence (heavy vehicles or buses) are permanently disqualified from driving.

Indications for defibrillator use

Primary prevention

Some patients can be identified as being at higher risk of sudden death. Primary prevention is considered in those who have had a previous myocardial infarction or non-ischaemic cardiomyopathy and depressed left ventricular systolic function (an ejection fraction of 35% or less).

The major primary prevention trials, including MADIT I and II, and MUSTT, showed that patients with implanted defibrillators had >50% improvement in survival compared with control patients, despite 75% of MADIT control patients being treated with the antiarrhythmic drug amiodarone. MADIT II randomised 1232 patients with any history of prior myocardial infarction and left ventricular dysfunction (ejection fraction <30%) to receive a defibrillator or to continue medical treatment and showed that patients with the device had a 31% reduction in risk of death. Although these results are good news clinically, they raise difficult questions about the potentially crippling economic impact of this added healthcare cost.

There is no single test that predicts which patients are at very high risk of sudden arrhythmic death. A number of parameters have been studied primarily looking at autonomic cardiac changes. T-wave electrical alternans (changes in T-wave microvoltage during exercise) demonstrates some promise at showing which patients are at low risk and who may not benefit from ICD implant.

Implantation is also appropriate for cardiac conditions with a known high risk of sudden death – long QT syndrome, hypertrophic cardiomyopathy, Brugada syndrome, arrhythmogenic right ventricular dysplasia and after repair of tetralogy of Fallot.

Secondary prevention

These are patients who present with a life-threatening arrhythmia and include the following:

- Successful resuscitation from cardiac arrest due to ventricular tachycardia or ventricular fibrillation, not due to a reversible cause (electrolyte imbalance, drugs)
- Spontaneous sustained ventricular tachycardia causing syncope or substantial haemodynamic compromise
- Sustained ventricular tachycardia without syncope or cardiac arrest in patients who have an associated reduction in ejection fraction (<35%)

If left untreated, these patients have a very high risk of arrhythmia recurrence and subsequent sudden death. Medical treatment with amiodarone is ineffective at significantly reducing sudden death. A meta-analysis of studies of implanted defibrillators for secondary prevention showed that they reduced the relative risk of death by 28%, almost entirely due to a 50% reduction in risk of sudden death.

Devices for heart failure

Heart failure

Many patients who present with ventricular arrhythmias have depressed left ventricular systolic function. Patients with heart failure, particularly ischaemic, are prone to sudden death. Some patients with impaired left ventricular function and clinical heart failure may benefit from the addition of a third pacing lead in the coronary sinus. This allows left ventricular pacing with resynchronisation of right and left ventricular contraction (biventricular pacing) (Figure 13.6). Indications for biventricular pacemakers/defibrillators include a broad QRS complex (>120 milliseconds with left bundle branch block on ECG), left ventricular systolic impairment and continued symptoms of heart failure despite optimal medical treatment (New York Heart Association class II–III). Biventricular pacing improves symptoms and confers a mortality benefit (CARE-HF study), particularly when combined with an ICD (COMPANION study).

Remote monitoring

Some types of ICD are capable of transmitting stored information via wireless or satellite to remote monitoring stations. The patient has a mobile phone type monitor at home or a transmitter attached to a landline. Information is transmitted on a regular basis, allowing the clinician to monitor the status of the device, arrhythmia type and frequency and any therapies given. Thus far devices cannot be reprogrammed remotely. The patient still has to attend the hospital if there are any significant problems, but it does allow some reassurance for minor issues. Other devices are capable of monitoring pulmonary impedance, which changes when the lungs

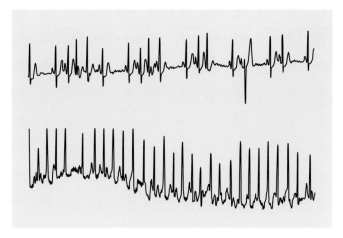

Figure 13.7 Continuous electrocardiogram showing sinus rhythm with frequent atrial extrasystoles (top) arising from the pulmonary veins degenerating into atrial fibrillation (bottom).

become oedematous thereby giving early warning of heart failure decompensation and allowing pre-emptive treatment.

Atrial flutter and fibrillation

Pacing to prevent atrial tachycardias, including atrial fibrillation, has been under intense scrutiny and although there is a small group of selected patients who may benefit, overall, pacing algorithms have not been proven effective (Figure 13.7). Clinically troublesome cases of atrial flutter or fibrillation can be treated with ablation. There was also a vogue for cardioversion with implantable atrial defibrillators but with the advent of successful ablative therapy this has also not gained widespread acceptance.

Future developments

With an ageing population, heart failure will be an increasing clinical problem and device implantation will increase. Studies looking at biventricular devices to prevent or slow down heart failure are currently underway and if proven will broaden the indication for these devices. Increased sophistication of remote monitoring may allow more patients to be managed at home.

Further reading

Connolly SJ, Hallstrom AP, Cappato R *et al*. Meta-analysis of the implantable cardioverter defibrillator secondary prevention trials. *Eur Heart J* 2000;**21**:2071–8.

Cooper RAS, Ideker RE. The electrophysiological basis for the prevention of tachyarrhythmias. In: Daubert JC, Prystowsky EN, Ripart A, eds. *Prevention of Tachyarrhythmias with Cardiac Pacing*. Armonk, NY: Futura Publishing, 1997;3–24.

Josephson ME. Supraventricular tachycardias. In: Bussy K, ed. *Clinical Cardiac Electrophysiology*. Philadelphia: Lea and Febiger, 1993;181–274.

Mirowski M, Mower MM, Staewen WS, Denniston RH, Mendeloff Al. The development of the transvenous automatic defibrillator. *Ann Intern Med* 1973;**129**:773–9.

O'Keefe DB. Implantable electrical devices for the treatment of tachyarrhythmias. In: Camm AJ, Ward DE, eds. *Clinical Aspects of Cardiac Arrhythmias*. London: Kluwer Academic Publishers, 1988;337–57.

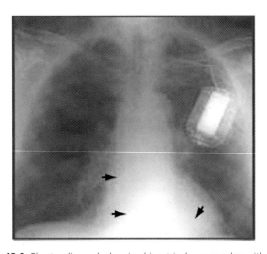

Figure 13.6 Chest radiograph showing biventricular pacemaker with leads in the right ventricle, right atrium and coronary sinus (arrows).

CHAPTER 14

Pacemakers for Bradycardia

Gerald C. Kaye

Princess Alexandra Hospital, Woolloongabba, Brisbane, QLD, Australia

---

OVERVIEW

- Patients with symptomatic bradycardias need assessment for a pacemaker
- Patients with pacemakers should be encouraged to live as normal a life as possible
- Any new swelling, redness, change in skin colour over the generator site or persistent pain requires urgent cardiological assessment
- Pacemaker checks are often required annually

Introduction

The implantation of the first self-contained pacemaker by Larsson and Elmqvist in 1958 paved the way for subsequent advances in pacing. Syncope due to slow heart rates could be prevented and patients' life expectancy could be extended. Early pacemakers were large and cumbersome and required thoracotomy and epicardial lead suturing. However, technological advances have allowed simpler implantation techniques. Better lead design, miniaturisation and improved battery technology allow units to function for many years without fail (Figure 14.1). As a result, pacing has become an accepted safe therapy in many clinical settings.

Technological advances

Although the first pacing devices were life-saving, a major limitation was that they were unable to sense the underlying cardiac rhythm and paced continuously. This meant that when bradycardia occurred, the pacemaker would take over the action of the heart but when the patient's rhythm had recovered, the device continued to pace. This reduced battery life considerably and also allowed the pacemaker to deliver a pacing output into the intrinsic T-wave – theoretically allowing ventricular arrhythmias to be initiated. These concerns led to the development of two basic advances that form the cornerstone of modern cardiac pacing – demand pacing and programmability.

ABC of Interventional Cardiology, 2nd edition.
© Ever D. Grech. Published 2011 Blackwell Publishing Ltd.

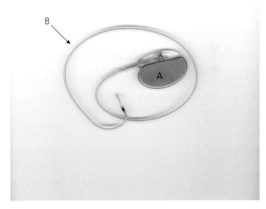

Figure 14.1 A pacemaker system consists of a hermetically sealed titanium can containing a battery power source together with electronic circuits to control timing and characteristics of the impulses it generates (A), and pacing lead (B). Modern devices are small, convenient, safe and reliable.

Demand pacing

The ability to sense spontaneous cardiac depolarisation and to inhibit pacemaker output allowed units to work only when required, thereby extending battery life. In patients with intermittent bradycardias, the pacemaker would be 'silent' when the heart's intrinsic rhythm was adequate but would 'cut in' when the heart rate fell to a predetermined level. For example, if the heart rate fell to less that 50 bpm, then the pacemaker could be programmed to deliver a pacing impulse (Figure 14.2a, b and c). Safety was also improved by avoiding pacing onto the intrinsic T-wave.

Programmability

Integrated circuits and microprocessors gave the first opportunities of externally altering pacemaker function, allowing adaptation to more physiological conditions. Initially, pacemakers could be programmed to alter their basic rate and pacing threshold (the amount of energy required to ensure the heart is always captured by the device). Devices are capable of testing lead integrity by measuring lead impedance using microvolt currents. Lead integrity is usually tested when the pacemaker is interrogated but modern devices now

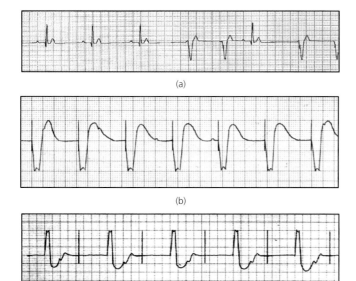

(a)

(b)

(c)

Figure 14.2 (a) An example of ventricular demand pacing (VVI). The first three beats are intrinsic. There is then slowing of the heart rate to a level below the programmed minimum pacing rate and the pacemaker delivers an impulse with capture (beats 4 and 5) until the intrinsic rate increases again (beat 6) which temporarily inhibits the pacemaker from delivering an impulse. (b) An example of continuous ventricular pacing. Characteristically the QRS complexes are broad with a left bundle branch block morphology. (c) An example of loss of capture. There are pacing spikes, which do not correspond to a QRS complex. The pacemaker provides an impulse but it does not capture the heart and therefore pacing is ineffective.

have the capacity for self-diagnostics (see subsequent sections) and can automatically test the leads on a regular basis. In modern basic devices, there are many programmable features including:

- The pacing rate
- The output of the device and pulse width
- Hysteresis (see the following section)

In more complex systems such as dual-chamber pacemakers or those with rate modulation, many additional features are programmable and will be discussed in the relevant section.

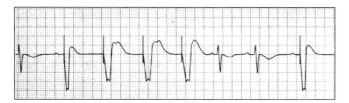

Figure 14.3 An example of hysteresis. The first beat is intrinsic. There is then slowing of the heart rate and the pacemaker is programmed to wait until the intrinsic heart rate falls below a pre-programmed level before it paces (second beat). The following three beats are also paced until the intrinsic heart rate recovers and the pacemaker stops pacing (it becomes inhibited – beats 6 and 7). The interval between the first intrinsic beat and the first paced beat is longer than the interval between the next three paced beats. The longer interval allows the underlying heart rhythm more time to recover before the pacemaker cuts in.

Hysteresis

Hysteresis allows the heart increased time for an intrinsic beat to come through, thereby extending device longevity and improving haemodynamics. The pacemaker is programmed to detect a fall in the heart rate to very low levels, for example 40/minute, but instead of pacing at the same rate, the device will pace at a higher more haemodynamically acceptable level, for example 70/minute. This allows more time for the intrinsic heart rate to come through, thereby preventing the pacemaker from pacing more than it needs to and extending battery life (Figure 14.3). It is also haemodynamically better for the patient allowing more time for the heart to fill.

Battery technology

Currently, lithium–iodide systems form the basic power supply of modern implantable devices. Pacemakers programmed to baseline settings would be expected to last around 7–8 years and some up to 12 years. More complex programmed functions will reduce device longevity.

Lead technology

Leads are a complex combination of an inner conductor coils allowing conduction of electrical impulses from the pacemaker to the endocardium and a plastic-type silicon or polyurethane material for insulation. This prevents ingress of body fluids into the electrodes and escape of electrical impulses to body fluids. As the heart beats 100,000 times a day, these leads must withstand all the sheer forces engendered by this recurrent movement and are thus constructed to prevent failure of either the conductor coils or the insulation. Lead failure is uncommon (<0.04% cases per year) and more commonly occurs at the site where the lead enters the venous circulation under the clavicle ('clavicular crush fracture', Figure 14.4).

Advances in lead technology include bipolar electrodes, better lead insulation, smaller lead size and improved lead tip technology such as laser-etched electrodes to increase surface area. Leads have either passive or active fixation. In passive fixation, the lead tip is designed to lodge itself within the endocardial trabeculations in the right ventricle (Figure 14.5b). The lead tip has an arrow head with tines made from silicone. These tines lock themselves into the trabeculations and with time become fibrosed to the endocardium. Passive fix leads are designed to be placed at the right ventricular

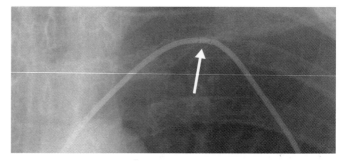

Figure 14.4 X-ray image of a single lead with a clear break in the outer insulation (white arrow) under the clavicle: a 'clavicular crush fracture'.

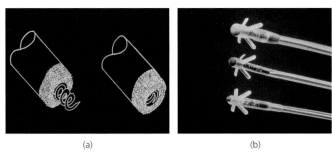

(a)   (b)

Figure 14.5 Pacing lead tips have various shapes to fit different modes of fixation. (a) Active fixation (screw-in) leads. (b) Passive fixation leads.

apex or right atrial appendage. They are designed to 'fall' into these positions easily and do not need much in the way of manipulation. An active fixation lead has a screw mechanism, which is actively screwed into the endocardium (Figure 14.5a). They are useful when a lead needs to be placed outside these areas, for example, in the right ventricular outflow area or in the high right atrium, particularly after cardiac surgery when the appendage has been amputated.

Better passive and active fixation techniques have been developed and include steroid-eluting tips to reduce the acute tissue reaction. Continuous audit has shown remarkable lead longevity with less than an average replacement of 1–2%.

Rate response

Early systems paced the heart at a constant rate irrespective of the patient's exercise requirements, causing breathlessness and fatigue. For example, the system would pace at 70/minute whether the patients were sitting or running. To allow the heart rate to increase when required and to a level commensurate with the desired exercise, sensors were developed, which detected changes in the patient's exercise requirements. One system uses a small crystal welded to the inside of the pacing can. Small vibrations in a crystal cause a tiny electric current (piezoelectric effect), which is detected and amplified. Changes in the rate of the signal reflect

the patient's exercise status. As the patient exercises, the rate of change in the signal from the crystal is fed back to a logic circuit in the integrated circuit, which then allows the pacing rate to increase accordingly. Other sensors use parameters such as changes in pulmonary minute ventilation, motion detectors (piezoelectric crystals, accelerometers), an assessment of cardiac contractility (impedance, QT sensor) changes in central body temperature and venous oxygen saturation. Sensor output can be tailored to each individual patient's need using bidirectional programmability. These sensors have revolutionised the use of pacemakers and allow them to behave in a more physiological way (Figure 14.6).

Pacemaker memory

Modern pacemakers have the capability of storing data. The percentage of pacing and the patient's own intrinsic rhythm are commonly stored parameters. This allows the pacemakers response to be tailored to an individual's requirement. If less pacing is required, the device can be programmed accordingly. Sensor information can also give data about how active the patient is and whether a more or less aggressive rate modulation is needed. Arrhythmias can also be stored, depending on where the lead is. In dual-chamber systems, both atrial and ventricular arrhythmias can be detected, increasing the pacemaker's diagnostic abilities (Figure 14.7). Some pacing systems allow the patient to trigger the storage of electrograms by placing a small magnet over the device. This enables symptoms to be related to the electrogram.

Clinical indications

The main indication for support pacing is bradycardia. The following clinical circumstances indicate permanent pacing:

1 Symptomatic sinus bradycardia – intermittent prolonged sinus pauses (usually in excess of 3 seconds) associated with syncope or presyncope.
2 Sick sinus syndrome – alternating episodes of atrial arrhythmias, such as atrial fibrillation or flutter with profound sinus bradycardias and/or long sinus pauses in excess of 3 seconds.

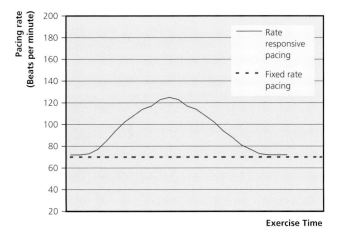

Figure 14.6 Rate-responsive pacing results in exercise-induced rise in the pacing rate that resembles a physiological response. The pacing rate declines following exercise cessation until it reaches the programmed basic rate.

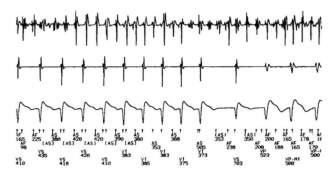

Figure 14.7 An example of the storage capabilities of current pacemakers. The above example shows the atrial electrogram on the upper trace, the ventricular in the middle and an equivalent of the surface electrocardiogram (ECG) on the lower. This recording confirms atrial fibrillation with a very rapid atrial rate and an irregular rapid ventricular response. The figures on the bottom correspond to the electrogram rate in milliseconds.

3 Heart block
  ◦ First degree – it is rare to require pacing for first-degree heart block. Pacing is only indicated if the patient is symptomatic, or for deemed haemodynamic benefit where persistent first-degree block is deleterious to the patient.
  ◦ Second-degree heart block – Mobitz type-II block mandates pacing. Mobitz type-I (Wenkebach) block rarely requires pacing.
  ◦ Acquired third-degree heart block (without a reversible cause; e.g. drugs toxicity).
  ◦ Congenital third-degree heart block – these patients are often asymptomatic but it is generally accepted now that a pacemaker is advised over the age of 50 years, irrespective of symptoms.
4 Carotid sinus hypersensitivity – a syndrome characterised by recurrent syncope/presyncope associated with the demonstration of a profound sinus pause (in excess of 5 seconds) during carotid sinus massage. This is an unusual syndrome, which requires careful patient assessment. Carotid sinus pressure is a relatively non-specific test and many patients have a sinus pause, which may or may not account for their symptoms. This is sometimes referred to as *reflex syncope* but must have a demonstrable bradycardic component.

Which type of pacemaker?

There are a number of different devices available (see Table 14.1). These are as follows:

- Single chamber ventricular demand pacemaker (VVI) – a single lead is placed in the right ventricle. The device is on demand. The following parameters are programmable: output, rate, pulse width and hysteresis.
- Single-chamber rate-responsive pacemaker (VVIR) – as above but has a rate sensor which responds to patients' exercise. Programmability is as above, plus the rate at which the sensor responds can be altered to make the device more or less aggressive to changes in the paced rate during exercise. Ideally, this can be tailored to each individual although in many cases an average rate (or slope) setting is sufficient.
- Dual-chamber pacemaker (DDD) – a two-lead device, one in the right atrium and one in the ventricle. These are sophisticated units, designed to more closely mimic the normal action of the heart beat. They have a plethora of programmable functions, which allow the device flexibility in managing individual patient's responses.
- Dual-chamber rate-responsive pacemaker (DDDR) – as above but with a rate sensor.

Pacemaker terminology

Table 14.1 denotes a coding for the different types of pacemakers currently available. This allows a shorthand description of each type. For example, a basic demand pacemaker which paces and senses the right ventricle is a VVI pacemaker. A demand pacemaker with a lead in the right ventricle capable of responding to exercise is a VVIR system. A DDDR pacemaker paces and senses in the atrium and ventricle and responds to exercise. The final column denotes more complex systems used in heart failure (cardiac resynchronisation) or dual-site atrial pacemaker.

Which pacemaker for which patient?

The current National Institute for Clinical Excellence (NICE) recommendations are as follows:

AAI or AAIR – used in the sick sinus syndrome where there is symptomatic bradycardia and no evidence of atrioventricular (AV) block. Rate response may be added if there is evidence of chronotropic incompetence (a lack of rate response with exercise).
VVI – this is rarely recommended nowadays.
VVIR – for patients with heart block in whom it is clinically felt that atrial transport may not make a significant difference. It should be used particularly when the underlying rhythm is atrial fibrillation where pacing in the atrium is not appropriate and ineffective.
DDD(R) – in patients with sinus rhythm and Mobitz type-II or third-degree heart block, either in isolation or in combination with the sick sinus syndrome. There will be clinical circumstances where patients' co-morbidity and frailty will influence the balance of risks and benefits in favour of a single-chamber ventricular device.

Complications

Acute
Procedural – the risk of a serious complication during pacemaker implantation is low. As the subclavian vein may need accessing with a needle puncture, a pneumothorax is the most common. The risk of a pneumothorax is 2%. Use of the cephalic vein (by dissecting directly onto the vein) removes this complication. Other complications are haematoma at the pacing site (2%), haemothorax (0.1%), damage to the brachial plexus or the chyle duct (rare). Perforation of the right ventricular apex with the pacing lead is probably relatively common but rarely causes serious trouble

Table 14.1 Coding for the different types of available pacemakers.

Position	I	II	III	IV	V
Category	Chamber paced	Chamber sensed	Response to sensing	Rate modulation	Multi-site pacing
	0 = None	0 = None	0 = None	0 = None	0 = None
	A = Atrium	A = Atrium	T = Triggered		A = Atrium
	V = Ventricle	V = Ventricle	I = Inhibited	R = Rate modulation	V = Ventricle
	D = Dual (A + V)	D = Dual (A + V)	D = Dual (T + I)		D = Dual (A + V)

(0.1%). Cardiac tamponade is rare. Acute infection within 48 hours is now very uncommon with the routine use of peri-procedural antibiotics. Lead displacement can occur particularly with active fixation atrial leads and accounts for 2–3% of complications.

Late
- Infection

  The most feared late complication is infection (Figure 14.8). Late infection occurs in 1–2% of cases. An infection of the system mandates removal, that is, the generator and the leads. Once the device has been implanted for over a year, removal of the leads can be difficult. It often requires the use of a cutting instrument to pull the lead from the endocardial surface and this carries small but serious risks. There is a 1–2% mortality risk and every case must be individually considered. Infection is an indication for mandatory lead removal.

- Generator/lead erosion (Figure 14.9)

  Lead and/or generator erosion occurs in 1–2% of cases and again once the generator or lead is exposed, superadded infection is usually guaranteed and the system requires removal. Although it is more commonly seen in very thin patients, it can occur at any time in any patient.

- Lead fracture

  Lead fracture is uncommon and often occurs under the clavicle as described above. Considering the mechanical stress the leads are under, lead fracture is relatively uncommon.

- Twiddler's syndrome

  This is an uncommon problem and occurs when patients intentionally or otherwise constantly rotate the generator within the pocket. This has the effect of twisting the leads within the heart and rarely can cause the leads to be pulled out of the endocardium (Figure 14.10a and b).

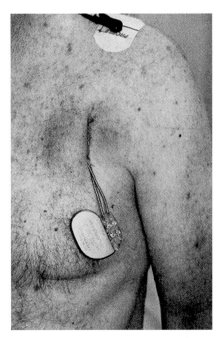

Figure 14.9 A dramatic example of a generator erosion. The skin over the generator has broken down and this allowed the generator and the leads to become exposed. There are no obvious signs of infection.

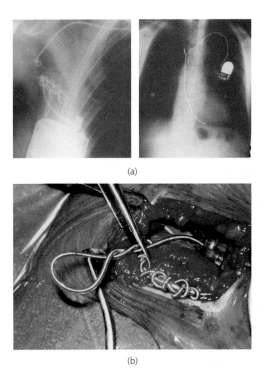

(a)

(b)

Figure 14.10 Twiddler's syndrome: (a) A chest X-ray on the right clearly showed that the lead is rotated and (b) at surgery the lead has become entwined in itself due to repeated rotation of the generator by the patient.

Pacing malfunction

Although cases have been described, it is very rare for pacemakers to fail suddenly. A common event is an increase in the pacing threshold usually within 2–3 months of the implant because of

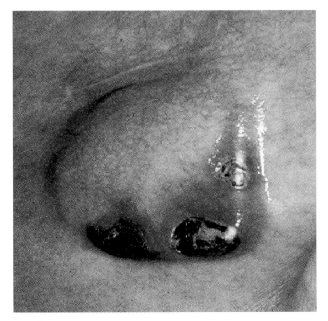

Figure 14.8 Generator site infection and subsequent erosion. The skin is thinned and erythematous and has broken down over the lower aspect of the can exposing the casing. This cannot be salvaged and needs removal.

fibrosis at the lead tip. This may lead to loss of capture and needs urgent reprogramming of the device to higher outputs. If this does not solve the problem, the lead may need to be replaced. Late increase in threshold after 6 months is rare. A recurrent issue is that of manufacturing faults. As these systems are so complex, faults in circuits do occur. Over time, every manufacturing company has been involved in recalling devices which, in some cases, need replacement, particularly if there is a battery fault.

Living with a pacemaker

- Driving – driving can be continued with a pacemaker, although the licensing authorities need to be informed. If syncope was present, then it is recommended that driving recommence 1 week after pacemaker implant. Heavy goods vehicle (HGV) drivers must inform the licensing authorities.
- Surgery – the issue with surgery is that of diathermy. The corporeal currents induced may temporarily inhibit pacemaker function. It is recommended that only bipolar diathermy (not unipolar) be used and if possible at least 10 cm away from the generator site. If this is not possible, the device should be protected by placing a magnet over the system during diathermy. This temporarily turns off the sensing circuits and forces the pacemaker to pace irrespective of the underlying rhythm. The patient will be protected when the magnet is on.
- Pregnancy – there is no contraindication to pregnancy by having a pacemaker already fitted and the risk pertain to the underlying cardiac condition. A normal delivery is possible with a pacemaker. The risks of diathermy during surgery, if required, are as above.
- Sex – the only limitation to normal sexual activities relates to the underlying heart disease.
- Travelling – airport security devices may be triggered by the device as may store security systems. It is advisable to inform the staff of the presence of a pacemaker. No damage will be done to the device provided the patient does not stand constantly within a magnetic field.

Pacemaker controversies

Although pacemakers are clearly life-saving and have been implanted for nearly 50 years, there is still controversy about where the best lead position should be. The favoured ventricular lead position has been the right ventricular apex. It is easily and readily accessible and lead technology has been designed to 'fall' into this position. However, over the past 10 years, it is clear that in some patients chronic right ventricular pacing may be deleterious, promoting heart failure and increasing mortality. This has been shown in patients where left ventricular systolic function is already impaired before pacing. It is understood that left ventricular

function is affected by right ventricular pacing and although biventricular pacing is good for certain types of heart failure, the optimal right-sided position remains unclear. Large-scale studies are currently underway to clarify this.

The present and future

Pacemaker technology is now very advanced. There are systems now which are able to continuously monitor lead integrity (impedance) and reprogram the device if there is a lead fracture.

Transtelephonic or a mobile phone wireless interrogation of pacemakers may allow interrogation from a distance. Very remote interrogation is possible with wireless system using a mobile phone or satellite networks, but as yet these system cannot be reprogrammed from a distance due to safety issues. In future, developments in global positioning systems (GPS) may allow remote interrogation and programming of pacemakers wherever patients are on the planet.

Conclusion

Technological developments over the past 50 years have confirmed reliable and effective cardiac pacing. A reduction in generator size, improved lead reliability and enhanced battery longevity have made pacemakers a routine part of cardiological treatment and has revolutionised many patients' lives. The future may promise genetic manipulation of the mammalian heart beat to a point where electronic devices like an implanted pacemaker will be obsolete. Until that time, a shiny can and some fancy integrated circuits will still be the main stay of patients with slow heartbeats.

Further reading

Gomez FP (ed.). *Cardiac Pacing*. Madrid, Spain: Grouz, 1985.

Gregoratos G, Abrams J, Epstein AE *et al.* ACC/AHA/NASPE 2002 guideline update for implantation of cardiac pacemakers and antiarrhythmia devices: summary article: a report of the American College of Cardiology/ American Heart Association Task Force on Practice Guidelines (ACC/ AHA/NASPE Committee to Update the 1998 Pacemaker Guidelines). *Circulation* 2002;**106**(16):2145–61.

NICE guidance for implantable pacemakers: TA88 bradycardia – dual chamber pacemakers: 2005. www.nice.org.uk.

Toff WD, Camm AJ, Skehan JD; United Kingdom Pacing and Cardiovascular Events Trial Investigators. Single-chamber versus dual-chamber pacing for high-grade atrioventricular block. *N Engl J Med* 2005;**353**(2): 145–55.

Wilkoff BL, Cook JR, Epstein AE *et al.* Dual-chamber pacing or ventricular backup pacing in patients with an implantable defibrillator: the Dual Chamber and VVI Implantable Defibrillator (DAVID) Trial. *JAMA* 2002;**288**(24):3115–23.

CHAPTER 15

Heart Failure, Dys-synchrony and Resynchronisation Therapy

Abdallah Al-Mohammad, Ever D. Grech and Jonathan Sahu

South Yorkshire Cardiothoracic Centre, Northern General Hospital, Sheffield, UK

OVERVIEW

- Patients with heart failure and severe left ventricular systolic dysfunction should be assessed for evidence of dys-synchrony

- Assessment of dys-synchrony depends on electrical and imaging criteria, based on the electrocardiogram (ECG) and echocardiography

- Cardiac resynchronisation therapy (CRT) is indicated in patients with heart failure due to left ventricular systolic dysfunction, who remain symptomatic on maximum medical therapy

- CRT leads to a reduction in symptoms and improvement in survival rate

- Patients at risk of life-threatening arrhythmias may also be considered for a CRT device which incorporates a defibrillator (CRT-D)

Heart failure

Heart failure is best defined as the syndrome of breathlessness, tiredness and fluid retention, caused by the inability of the dysfunctional heart to deliver blood and oxygen in quantities commensurate with the requirements of the metabolising tissues.

Types of heart failure

Heart failure can be caused by dysfunction of the myocardium (majority of the patients), the valves, the pericardium, the endocardium or the conduction system. Of the heart failure caused by myocardial dysfunction, 54% of patients will have impairment of myocardial contraction which is referred to as *systolic dysfunction* (Figures 15.1 and 15.2). The remainder can be mainly described as having *heart failure with preserved left ventricular ejection fraction* (LVEF). The latter remains a controversial term as there is no agreement on the level of ejection fraction above which it can be labelled as preserved. In addition, there are varying explanations to this form of heart failure, and some claim that there is impairment of contraction on the longitudinal axis of the left ventricle.

Prevalence of heart failure

Heart failure is the new cardiovascular epidemic. Its increasing prevalence is multi-factorial: the improved survival of myocardial infarction, the improved longevity of sufferers of chronic diseases likely to result in heart failure (such as hypertension and diabetes mellitus) and the increased longevity of the population in general. Heart failure affects 2% of the population, rising with age to 10–20% in the elderly.

Therapeutic interventions in heart failure

Until 1986, there were three surgical interventions likely to transform the outlook of some patients with heart failure. These were valve surgery, coronary artery bypass surgery in patients with severe left ventricular systolic dysfunction and three-vessel disease and heart transplantation.

Since then, the therapeutic armamentarium has expanded, especially in the management of left ventricular systolic dysfunction. These include angiotensin-converting enzyme inhibitors (ACEIs), angiotensin-II receptor (type-1) blockers (ARBs), β-receptor blockers, aldosterone antagonists and the combination of hydralazine and nitrates.

Several new surgical interventions including mitral valve repair and left ventricular remodelling are other additions to the non-pharmacological interventions in heart failure. In addition, there are pacing interventions including cardiac resynchronisation therapy (CRT) and implantable cardioverter defibrillators (ICD).

Dys-synchrony

Dys-synchrony is best defined as the presence of segments within the same pumping cavity that are not contracting and relaxing simultaneously. In a dys-synchronous left ventricle, the delay could be such that segments of the left ventricular wall will be relaxing while others are starting to contract. This carries increased importance when the left ventricle is dilated and significantly impaired. It is usually associated with dysfunction of the mitral valve, caused by dys-synchrony of the segments to which the papillary muscles are attached. Thus, the mitral valve becomes regurgitant, even if its leaflets are normal. In a subgroup of these patients with significant delays in contraction, the mitral regurgitation could even occur in the diastolic phase – *diastolic mitral regurgitation.*

ABC of Interventional Cardiology, 2nd edition.
© Ever D. Grech. Published 2011 Blackwell Publishing Ltd.

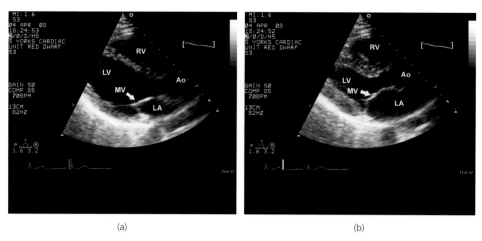

(a)   (b)

Figure 15.1 Example of normal left ventricular contraction in an adult. The echocardiographic images are acquired in the parasternal long axis view in diastole (a) and in systole (b). Note that the contraction results in a significant reduction of the left ventricular volume. LV, left ventricle; LA, left atrium; MV, mitral valve; Ao, aorta; RV, right ventricle.

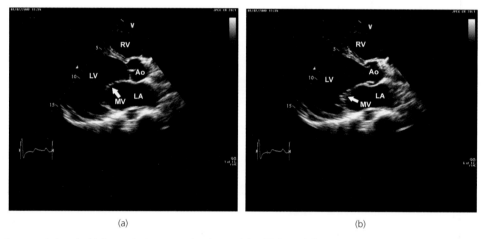

(a)   (b)

Figure 15.2 Example of a severely impaired left ventricular contraction in an adult with heart failure. Images were acquired in the parasternal long axis view in diastole (a) and in systole (b). In contrast to the appearance of normal left ventricular function seen in Figure 15.1, note that the contraction does not result in a significant reduction of the left ventricular volume. LV, left ventricle; LA, left atrium; MV, mitral valve; Ao, aorta; RV, right ventricle.

Dys-synchrony may exist between atrial and ventricular contraction (*atrio-ventricular dys-synchrony*), between the left and the right ventricles (*interventricular dys-synchrony* or *mechanical delay*) and within the left ventricle (*intraventricular dys-synchrony*).

One potential solution for dys-synchrony is to pace the left and right ventricles simultaneously, allowing the various parts of the left ventricle to contract with less delay. As a result, several of the characteristics of dys-synchrony may be ameliorated or even corrected and this is referred to as *cardiac resynchronisation therapy* (CRT).

The aims of CRT are to reduce the left ventricular size, reduce mitral regurgitation and improve the efficiency of the left ventricle as a pump. Several clinical trials have demonstrated that CRT can reduce morbidity. Furthermore, the CARE-HF trial demonstrated for the first time that CRT resulted in a significant reduction in mortality.

The pacing method to achieve this is by multi-site pacing. This involves pacing the left ventricle via the coronary sinus tributaries, the right ventricle at the apex or even better at the septum, as well as the right atrium (Figures 15.3 and 15.4). Where pacing

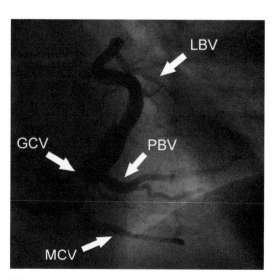

Figure 15.3 Coronary sinus venogram (antero-posterior projection) showing guide catheter tip at the ostium of the great cardiac vein (GCV). LBV, lateral branch vein; PBV, posterior branch vein; MCV, middle cardiac vein branch.

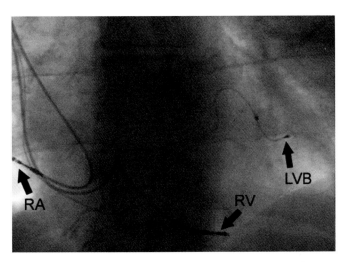

Figure 15.4 Final placement of the three cardiac resynchronisation therapy (CRT) leads (antero-posterior projection). RA, right atrial lead tip in right atrium; RV, right ventricular lead tip in right ventricular apex; LVB, left ventricular lead tip in lateral branch vein.

via the coronary sinus proves to be either difficult or impossible, the alternative is to surgically attach a left ventricular epicardial lead, while the other leads are inserted transvenously. The implanted pacing device has the CRT-P acronym (where P stands for pacing).

As these patients may also be at risk of life-threatening arrhythmias, a CRT device may incorporate a defibrillator (CRT-D), which may be considered in those who separately fulfil the criteria for the use of an *implantable cardioverter defibrillator* (ICD).

Diagnosis of cardiac dys-synchrony

Widening of the QRS complex on the electrocardiogram has been used as a marker of dys-synchrony and may be associated with a worse prognosis. Even in the absence of heart failure, the widening of QRS complexes to beyond 120 milliseconds, such as in left bundle branch block, may be associated with visible dys-synchrony of the left ventricle. The wider the QRS complex, the higher the likelihood for the left ventricle to be dys-synchronous. A QRS complex longer than 150 milliseconds is sufficient to identify mechanical dys-synchrony in a patient with heart failure and left ventricular systolic dysfunction. In patients with heart failure and a QRS complex measuring 120–149 milliseconds, there is a need to demonstrate echocardiographic evidence of mechanical dys-synchrony before applying CRT.

The diagnosis is relevant in patients presenting with symptomatic heart failure, New York Heart Association (NYHA) class II–IV (this is wider than the current NICE guidelines as there is recent evidence to suggest that patients with NYHA class II would benefit from CRT), who have evidence of left ventricular systolic dysfunction. The latter can be diagnosed by echocardiography showing regional or global impairment of contraction (Figure 15.2). The impairment needs to be severe for the patient to benefit from CRT.

Patients are more likely to benefit from CRT in the presence of secondary mitral regurgitation (caused by the dilatation of the mitral valve annulus or the distortion of the mitral valve leaflets

and/or the mitral valve apparatus, due to the left ventricular dysfunction). The likelihood of a positive response to CRT is also increased if the secondary mitral regurgitation can be demonstrated to be due to the effect of dys-synchrony on the mitral apparatus.

Echocardiographic evidence for mechanical dys-synchrony

Despite the doubts raised by the PROSPECT study on the validity of echocardiography in predicting the response to CRT, this remains one of the methods used to select patients for CRT. The PROSPECT study looked at the identification of dys-synchrony by echocardiography. It concluded that there was not a single echocardiographic parameter that was sufficient to identify patients with dys-synchrony.

However, while no single echocardiographic marker could be regarded as sufficient to make the diagnosis in the study cohort, the diagnosis has to be considered in the presence of several signs and parameters. In addition, there were some methodological concerns with the study.

Two-dimensional echocardiography provides the visual evidence of dys-synchrony, but this needs to be objectively measured using one of the following methods:

1 On cross-sectional images (M-mode) of the left ventricle, a delay between the peak of contraction between the anterior wall and the infero-posterior wall of over 130 milliseconds defines intraventricular dys-synchrony (Figure 15.5).

2 On two-dimensional echocardiography, the application of tissue Doppler imaging (TDI) can detect with high sensitivity the timing of peak shortening, especially on the longitudinal axis (see normal TDI pattern in Figure 15.6 and abnormal patterns in Figure 15.7). The delay from the onset of the QRS complex to the peak of contraction (S-wave on TDI) can be measured for several walls of the left ventricle. The most important (for our ability to correct them by CRT) are the differences between the lateral wall and the septum. Others include the anterior and the inferior walls. A difference in the delay to peak contraction between two walls of more than 40 milliseconds identifies dys-synchrony in the left ventricle – *intraventricular dys-synchrony* (Figure 15.7). Some studies indicate that elevating the threshold to 65 milliseconds improves this sign's specificity (likelihood of a positive response to CRT).

3 Another parameter is the difference in the delay to onset or peak ejection time between the two ventricles. This is measured by applying flow Doppler to the aortic and pulmonary valves (Figure 15.8). When the difference between the delay from the onset of QRS complex and the onset of ejection (or its peak) in the aortic and pulmonary arteries is more than 40 milliseconds, *interventricular dys-synchrony* is said to be present (Figure 15.9).

Using the same principles of TDI, newer echocardiographic machines are capable of simultaneously interrogating several walls, thus measuring the TDI of all these walls during the same myocardial contraction. The display of the results is usually by simultaneous curves that are superimposed unless there was dys-synchrony where

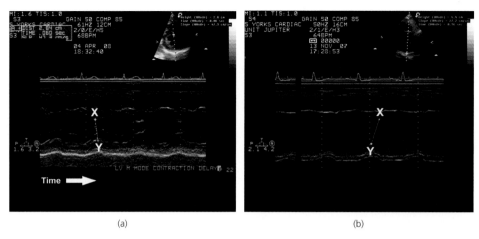

(a)   (b)

Figure 15.5 Two examples of measurement of intraventricular contraction delay on M-mode echocardiography. The delay is the time difference between the peak contraction of the anterior wall (point X) and the peak contraction of the inferior wall (point Y). The image is produced by applying an M-mode cross section through a short axis view of the left ventricle. (a) The measured time delay of 60 milliseconds is within normal limits (<130 milliseconds) in an adult with normal left ventricular contraction. (b) An abnormally long time delay in a patient with heart failure and left ventricular dys-synchrony (>130 milliseconds).

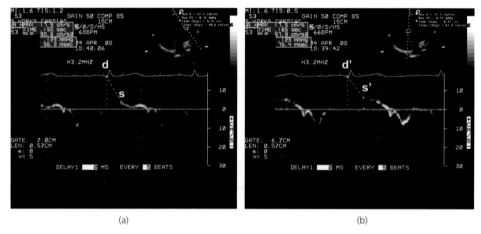

(a)   (b)

Figure 15.6 Examples of tissue Doppler imaging (TDI) assessment of the mechanical synchrony of left ventricular contraction in a normal adult. Two walls are said to be synchronous if the difference between the time delays to peak contraction of these two walls is <40 milliseconds. The delay is the interval between the onset of depolarisation (at the beginning of the QRS complex on the electrocardiogram (ECG)) and the peak of contraction (represented by the peak of the S-wave on TDI). (a) The time delay of 150 milliseconds in the lateral wall between the onset of depolarisation (d) and the peak of contraction (s). (b) The time delay of 165 milliseconds in the septal wall between the onset of depolarisation (d') and the peak of contraction (s'). Note that the time difference is 15 milliseconds, which is normal.

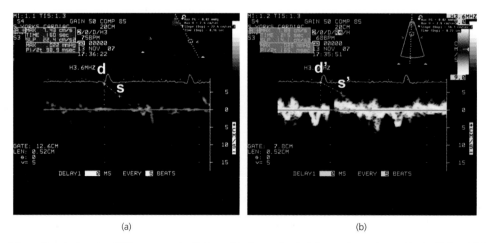

(a)   (b)

Figure 15.7 Example of tissue Doppler imaging (TDI) assessment of intraventricular mechanical dys-synchrony in a patient with heart failure. The two walls are said to be dys-synchronous if the difference between the time delays to peak contraction of these two walls is over 40 milliseconds. The delay is the interval between the onset of depolarisation (at the beginning of the QRS complex on the electrocardiogram (ECG)) and the peak of contraction (represented by the peak of the S-wave on TDI). (a) The delay (160 milliseconds) in the lateral wall between the onset of depolarisation (d) and the peak of contraction (s). (b) The delay (215 milliseconds) in the septal wall between the onset of depolarisation (d') and the peak of contraction (s'). Note that the time difference is 55 milliseconds, which is abnormal.

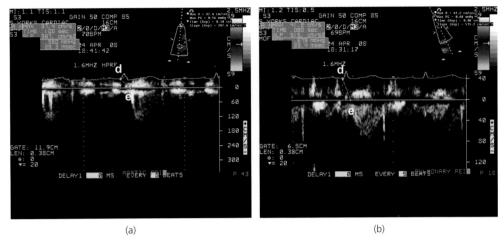

(a)   (b)

Figure 15.8 The interventricular mechanical delay in a normal adult. This is the difference between the aortic pre-ejection interval (PEI) and the pulmonary PEI. The difference between the two does not normally exceed 40 milliseconds. The PEI is the time delay between the onset of depolarisation (onset of QRS complex on the electrocardiogram (ECG)) (d) and the onset of ejection on Doppler flow (e). (a) The PEI of the aorta (100 milliseconds). (b) The PEI of the pulmonary artery (80 milliseconds). Note that the time difference is 20 milliseconds, which is normal.

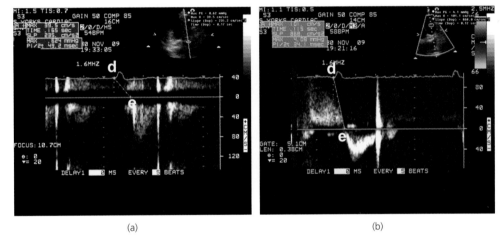

(a)   (b)

Figure 15.9 Abnormal interventricular mechanical delay (interventricular dys-synchrony) in a patient with heart failure. This is based on the difference between the aortic pre-ejection interval (PEI) and the pulmonary PEI being over 40 milliseconds. The PEI is the time delay between the onset of depolarisation (onset of QRS complex on the electrocardiogram (ECG)) (d) and the onset of ejection on Doppler flow (e). (a) The PEI of the aorta (165 milliseconds). (b) The PEI of the pulmonary artery (115 milliseconds). Note that the time difference is 50 milliseconds, which is abnormal.

the curves will be deviated from each other. This will allow us to more easily discern the differences in the time-to-peak contraction of different walls.

Other more specialised techniques that follow the same principles above may also be used.

Guidelines from National Institute of Health and Clinical Excellence (NICE)

In recognition of the difficulties in identifying the patients most likely to benefit from CRT, the National Institute of Health and Clinical Excellence (NICE) has suggested the following guidelines.

Patients with heart failure due to severe left ventricular systolic dysfunction (LVEF <35%), who have severe symptoms (NYHA class ≥III) and whose electrocardiogram shows sinus rhythm and prolonged QRS complexes ≥120 milliseconds, should be considered for CRT if they have either

1 QRS complexes ≥150 milliseconds, or
2 QRS complexes = 120–149 milliseconds and echocardiographic evidence of mechanical dys-synchrony as defined above.

These guidelines are reviewed regularly with the emergence of new evidence. The next review by NICE is due for release in the near future.

Further reading

Abraham WT, Fisher WG, Smith AL *et al.* Cardiac resynchronization in chronic heart failure. *N Engl J Med* 2002;**346**:1845–53.

Bonow RO, Udelson JE. Left ventricular diastolic dysfunction as a cause of congestive heart failure. Mechanisms and management. *Ann Intern Med* 1992;**117**(6):502–10.

Bristow MR, Saxon LA, Boehmer J *et al.* Cardiac-resynchronization therapy with or without an implantable defibrillator in advanced chronic heart failure. *N Engl J Med* 2004;**350**:2140–50.

Cardiac resynchronisation therapy for the treatment of heart failure. NICE technology appraisal guidance 120. http://www.nice.org.uk/nicemedia/pdf/TA120Guidance.pdf.

Cleland JG, Daubert JC, Erdmann E *et al.* The effect of cardiac resynchronization on morbidity and mortality in heart failure. *N Engl J Med* 2005;**352**:1539–49.

Flachskampf FA, Voigt J-U. Echocardiographic methods to select candidates for cardiac resynchronization therapy. *Heart* 2006;**92**:424–9.

Young JB, Abraham WT, Smith AL *et al.* Combined cardiac resynchronization and implantable cardioversion defibrillation in advanced chronic heart failure: the MIRACLE ICD trial. *J Am Med Assoc* 2003;**289**: 2685–94.

Yu CM, Abraham WT, Bax J *et al.* Predictors of Response to Cardiac Resynchronization Therapy (PROSPECT) – study design. *Am Heart J* 2005;**149**:600–5.

CHAPTER 16

Interventional Paediatric Cardiology

Damien Kenny[1] *and Kevin P. Walsh*[2]

[1]Bristol Royal Hospital for Children, Bristol, UK
[2]Our Lady's Hospital for Sick Children, Dublin, UK

> **OVERVIEW**
>
> - Experience is evolving, and ongoing modifications to devices and equipment are aimed at abolition of the haemodynamic abnormality with minimal long-term impact on the heart and great vessels
> - The heterogeneous nature of the patient population and heart anatomy requires an individualised approach to each patient
> - Meticulous pre-procedural preparation with a flexible approach to unforeseen intra-operative events is essential
> - Future directions include biodegradable devices, percutaneous valve implantation and greater collaboration with surgeon and interventionalist in the hybrid approach to challenging defects

Interventional paediatric cardiology mainly involves dilatation of stenotic vessels or valves and occlusion of abnormal communications. Advances in imaging, techniques such as hybrid procedures and equipment including biodegradable devices and stents, are driving the pursuit of minimally invasive correction or palliation. These avoid the long-term sequelae of fixed foreign bodies within the heart and major arteries.

Basic techniques

General anaesthesia or sedation is essential in children. Although most procedures start with femoral access, the choice of percutaneous access is based on the individual anatomy and procedures and may include transhepatic or umbilical approach. Haemodynamic measurements and angiograms may further delineate the anatomy or lesion severity. A catheter is passed across the stenosis or abnormal communication. A guidewire is then passed through the catheter to provide a track over which therapeutic devices are delivered. Balloon catheters are threaded directly, whereas stents and occlusion devices are protected or constrained within long plastic sheaths.

Dilatations

Septostomy

Balloon atrial septostomy, introduced by Rashkind 35 years ago, improves mixing of oxygenated and deoxygenated blood in patients with transposition physiology or in those requiring venting of an atrium with restricted outflow (Figure 16.1). In slightly older infants, the atrial septum is much tougher, and creation of a defect may require cutting the atrial septum with a blade.

Balloon valvuloplasty
Pulmonary valve stenosis

Balloon valvuloplasty has become the treatment of choice for pulmonary valve stenosis in all age groups. It relieves the stenosis by tearing the valve, and the resultant pulmonary regurgitation is well tolerated (Figure 16.2). Surgery is used only for dysplastic valves, especially in patients with Noonan's syndrome, who have small valve rings and require a patch to enlarge the annulus.

Valvuloplasty is especially useful in neonates with critical (duct-dependent) pulmonary stenosis, where surgery carries a high mortality. In neonates with membranous pulmonary atresia, valvuloplasty can still be done by first perforating the pulmonary valve with a hot wire using radiofrequency energy followed by balloon dilatation. Pulmonary valvuloplasty may improve cyanotic spells in patients with tetralogy of Fallot, although subvalvar muscular obstruction is not significantly affected by balloon dilatation.

Aortic valve stenosis

Unlike in adults, aortic valve stenosis in children is non-calcific and maybe treated effectively by balloon dilatation. A balloon size close to the annulus diameter is chosen, as overdilatation (routinely done in pulmonary stenosis) can result in substantial aortic regurgitation. The balloon is usually introduced retrogradely via the femoral artery and passed across the aortic valve. Injection of adenosine or rapid ventricular pacing avoids balloon ejection by powerful left ventricular contraction.

In neonates with critical aortic stenosis and poor left ventricular function, the balloon can be introduced in an antegrade fashion, via the femoral vein and across the interatrial septum through the patent foramen ovale. This reduces the risk of femoral artery thrombosis and perforation of the soft neonatal aortic valve

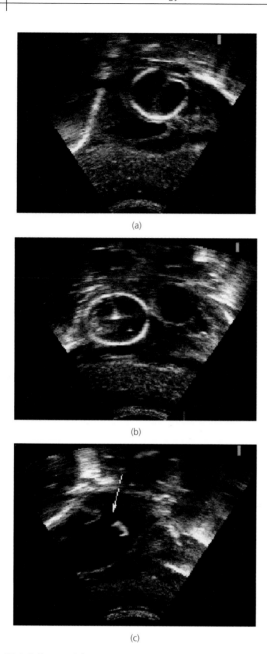

(a)

(b)

(c)

Figure 16.1 Balloon atrial septostomy. Under echocardiographic control in a neonate with transposition of the great arteries, a balloon septostomy catheter has been passed via the umbilical vein, ductus venosus, inferior vena cava and right atrium and through the patent foramen ovale into the left atrium. The balloon is inflated in the left atrium (a) and jerked back across the atrial septum into the right atrium (b). This manoeuvre tears the atrial septum to produce an atrial septal defect (arrow, (c)) with improved mixing and arterial saturations.

leaflets by guidewires. Long-term result of aortic valve dilatation in neonates is similar to surgery, with approximately 50% requiring reintervention at 5 years.

Angioplasty

Balloon dilatation for coarctation of the aorta is used for both native coarctation and re-coarctation. Neonates in whom the ductal tissue forms a sling around the arch have a good initial response to

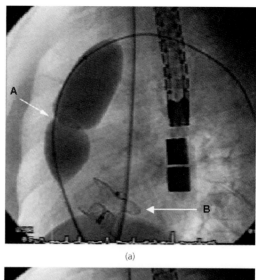

(a)

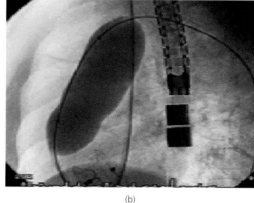

(b)

Figure 16.2 Balloon pulmonary valvuloplasty. A large valvuloplasty balloon is inflated across a stenotic pulmonary valve, which produces a waist-like balloon indentation (A, (a)). Further inflation of the balloon abolishes the waist (b). This patient had previously undergone closure of a mid-muscular ventricular septal defect with a drum-shaped Amplatzer ventricular septal defect occluder (B, (a)). A transoesophageal echocardiogram probe is also visible.

dilatation but a high restenosis rate, and surgery maybe a preferred option. Older children have a good response to balloon dilatation; however, overdilatation may result in the formation of an aneurysm, and stenting is preferable. Angioplasty is also used for pulmonary artery and pulmonary vein stenosis. In cases with significant scar, tissue-cutting balloons with longitudinally mounted microsurgical blades have been employed.

Stents

The problems of vessel recoil or dissection have been addressed by the introduction of endovascular stents. This development has been particularly important for patients with pulmonary artery stenoses, especially those who have undergone corrective surgery, for whom repeat surgery can be disappointing. Most stents are balloon expandable and can be further expanded after initial deployment with a larger balloon to keep up with a child's growth.

Results from stent implantation for pulmonary artery stenosis have been good, with sustained increases in vessel diameter, distal

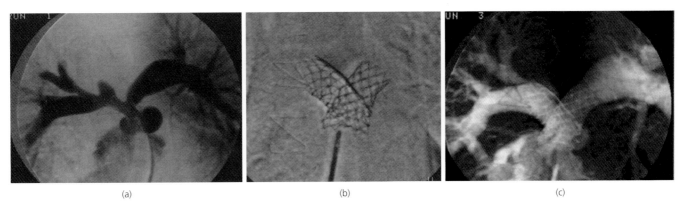

(a) (b) (c)

Figure 16.3 Pulmonary artery stenting. A child with previously repaired tetralogy of Fallot has severe stenosis at the junction of the right and left branch pulmonary arteries with the main pulmonary artery (a). Two stents have been inflated simultaneously across the stenoses in a criss-cross arrangement (b). Angiography shows complete relief of the stenoses (c).

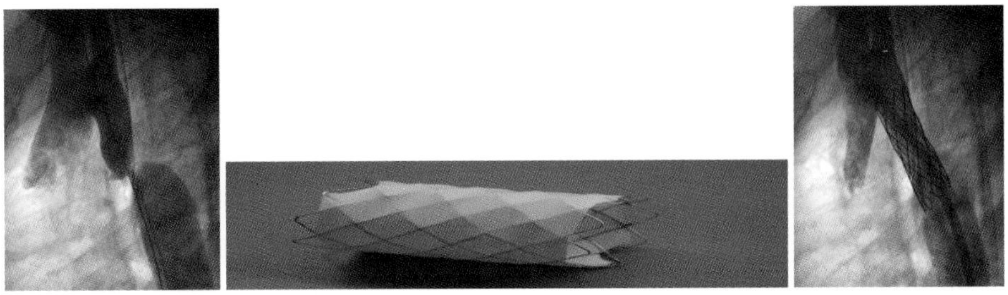

Figure 16.4 Near atretic coarctation of the aorta and stenting with a covered stent. The narrowed segment (a) is crossed with a wire and a covered stent (b) is inflated on a balloon catheter across the coarctation with excellent result as seen in (c). This patient had undergone previous surgical repair with a subclavian flap (left subclavian not seen).

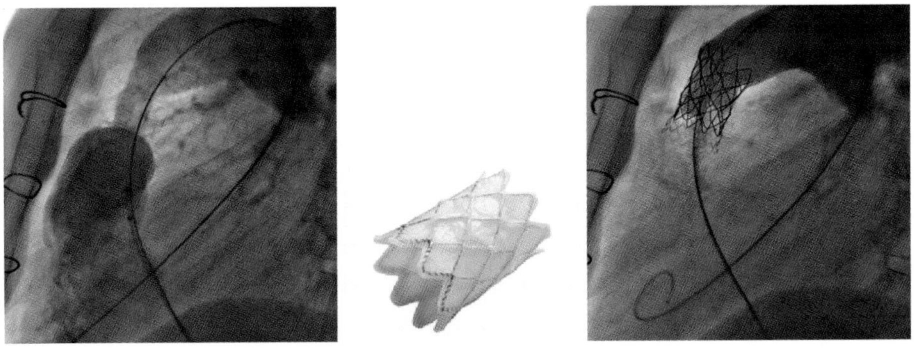

(a) (b) (c)

Figure 16.5 Percutaneous pulmonary valve implantation. A patient with previous right ventricle to pulmonary artery conduit has developed severe conduit stenosis (a). The Medtronic Melody valve (b) is inserted via the groin crimped onto a balloon catheter. In the case shown opposite, the right ventricular outflow tract has been stented as part of the same procedure to provide support for the new pulmonary valve. The result is a non-stenotic, competent valve without the need for surgery (c).

(a) (b) (c)

perfusion and gradient reduction (Figure 16.3). Complications consist of stent misplacement and embolisation, in-situ thrombosis and vessel rupture.

Stents are increasingly used to treat native coarctation and re-coarctation in older children and adolescents (Figure 16.4). Graded dilatation may be required to avoid overdistension and possible aneurysm formation, although development of covered stents may reduce the consequences of aneurysms. Self-expanding covered stents have been used in aneurysm formation without re-coarctation and also to occlude conduit dehiscence in those with a total cavopulmonary connection.

Stenting of the arterial duct in duct-dependent congenital heart disease has re-emerged following initially disappointing results. This provides an alternative to surgical arterio-pulmonary shunting in selected cases.

Percutaneous pulmonary valve replacement is evolving and well over 1000 cases have now been performed. A bovine jugular vein valve is sutured to the inner aspect of a large stent, which is crimped onto a balloon delivery system and then expanded in an outflow conduit previously placed surgically. Some degree of calcification of the conduit is necessary to ensure that the stent is wedged in place, and prior stenting of the right ventricular outflow tract maybe necessary (Figure 16.5).

Occlusions

Transcatheter occlusion of intracardiac and extracardiac communications has been revolutionised by the development of the Amplatzer devices. These are made from a cylindrical Nitinol wire mesh and formed by heat treatment into different shapes. A sleeve with a female thread on the proximal end of the device allows attachment of a delivery cable with a male screw. The attached device can then be pulled and pushed into the loader and delivery sheath,

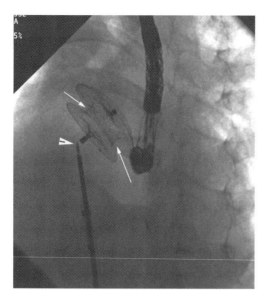

Figure 16.6 Cineframe showing the three components of the Amplatzer atrial septal defect occluder – a left atrial disc, central stent (arrows) and a right atrial disc. The device has just been unscrewed from the delivery wire, and the male screw on the delivery wire can be seen (arrowhead).

respectively. A family of devices has been produced to occlude ostium secundum atrial septal defects, patent foramen ovale, patent ductus arteriosus and both muscular and perimembranous ventricular septal defects. A generic vascular plug has also been developed and used to occlude venous collaterals and coronary artery fistulae.

A range of other devices have since become available aiming to achieve total occlusion with low profile and minimal long-term impact on the heart. The ultimate goal is a fully biodegradable device and although not yet achieved, the new Biostar atrial septal defect device consisting of purified acellular porcine intestinal collagen mounted on a double umbrella frame has been implanted in a number of patients.

Atrial septal defects

The Amplatzer atrial septal defect occluder has the shape of two saucers connected by a central stent-like cylinder that varies in

diameter from 4 mm to 40 mm to allow closure of both small and large atrial septal defects. Very large secundum atrial septal defects with incomplete margins (other than at the aortic end of the defect) may require a surgically placed patch.

Choice of occluder diameter is usually based on sizing of the defect with a compliant balloon catheter. The occluder is then introduced into the left atrium via a long transvenous sheath. The left atrial disc of the occluder is extruded and pulled against the defect. The sheath is then pulled back to deploy the rest of the device (central waist and right atrial disc) and released after its placement is assessed by transoesophageal or intracardiac echocardiography. The defect is closed by the induction of thrombosis on three polyester patches sewn into the device and covered by neocardia within 2 months. Aspirin is usually given for 6 months and clopidrogrel for 6–12 weeks.

Worldwide, several thousand patients have had their atrial septal defects closed with Amplatzer devices, with high occlusion rates (Figures 16.6 and 16.7). Complications are unusual and consist of device migration (<1%), transient arrhythmias (1–2%) and, rarely, thrombus formation with cerebral thromboembolism or aortic erosion with tamponade. Transcatheter occlusion is now the treatment of choice for patients with suitable atrial septal defects.

Patent foramen ovale

Numerous patent foramen ovale closure devices are available and have been implanted in children with cryptogenic stoke and right-to-left shunt at atrial level (Figure 16.8). Randomised trials in adults comparing efficacy of closure in preventing recurrence versus medical treatment have struggled to recruit adequate numbers.

Patent ductus arteriosus

Although premature babies and small infants with a large patent ductus arteriosus are still treated surgically, older infants and children with a patent ductus arteriosus are treated by transcatheter coil occlusion. This technique has been highly successful at closing small defects, but when the minimum diameter is >3 mm, multiple and larger diameter coils are required, which prolongs the procedure (Figure 16.9). The Amplatzer patent ductus arteriosus plug, which

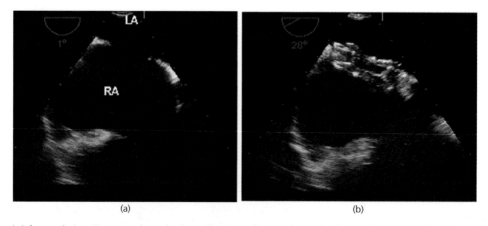

(a)   (b)

Figure 16.7 Atrial septal defect occlusion. Transoesophageal echocardiograms of an atrial septal defect before (a) and after (b) occlusion with an Amplatzer atrial septal defect device. The three components of the device are easily seen. LA, left atrium; RA, right atrium.

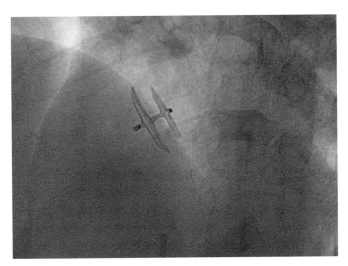

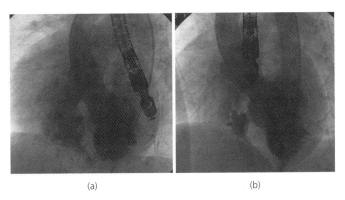

(a)   (b)

Figure 16.11 Transcatheter closure of a mid-muscular ventricular septal defect. A left ventriculogram shows substantial shunting of dye through a defect in the mid-muscular ventricular septum (a). After placement of an Amplatzer muscular ventricular septal defect device, a repeat left ventriculogram shows only a small amount of shunting through the device (b), which ceased after 3 months.

Figure 16.8 Patent foramen ovale closure. A cineframe of an implanted Amplatzer patent foramen ovale device shows that it differs from the atrial septal defect device in not having a central stent. Its right atrial disc is larger than the left atrial disc and faces in a concave direction towards the atrial septum.

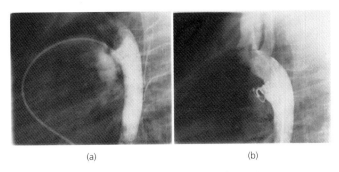

(a)   (b)

Figure 16.9 Coil occlusion of a patent ductus arteriosus. An aortogram performed via the transvenous approach shows dye shunting through the small conical patent ductus arteriosus into the pulmonary artery (a). After placement of multiple coils, a repeat aortogram shows no residual shunting (b).

has a mushroom-shaped Nitinol frame stuffed with polyester, is used for occluding larger defects (Figure 16.10). The occlusion rates are close to 100%.

Ventricular septal defects

Occlusion devices are especially useful for multiple congenital muscular ventricular septal defects, which can be difficult to correct

surgically. The Amplatzer occluder device has a drum-like shape and is deployed through long sheaths with relatively small diameter (Figure 16.11).

Such devices have also been used to occlude perimembranous defects, although in this location they can interfere with aortic valve function. An Amplatzer device with eccentric discs, which should avoid interference with adjacent valves, has recently been introduced (Figure 16.12). This has two discs connected by a short cylindrical waist. The device is eccentric, with the left ventricular disc having no margin superiorly, where it could come near the aortic valve, and a longer margin inferiorly to hold it on the left ventricular side of the defect. The end screw of the device has a flat portion, which allows it to be aligned with a precurved pusher catheter. This pusher catheter then extrudes the eccentric left ventricular disc from the specially curved sheath with its longer margin orientated inferiorly in the left ventricle. There have been concerns regarding early and late complete heart block presumably due to interference with the conduction system and rates of 5% are quoted.

Transcatheter occlusion has also been used to treat ventricular septal defects in adults who have had a myocardial infarction, and a specific occluder has been introduced. It differs from the infant device in having a 10-mm long central stent to accommodate the thicker adult interventricular septum. It offers an alternative to surgery where mortality rates are high, and initial results are promising.

Figure 16.10 Transcatheter plugging of a large patent ductus arteriosus. An aortogram shows a large tubular patent ductus arteriosus with a large shunt of dye from the aorta to the pulmonary artery (a). An Amplatzer plug is deployed in the defect, still attached to its delivery wire (b). A repeat aortogram after release of the device shows no significant residual shunting (c).

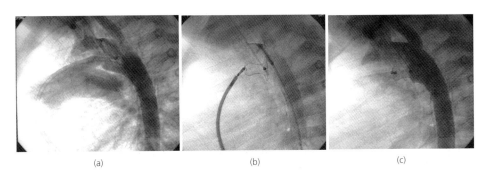

(a)   (b)   (c)

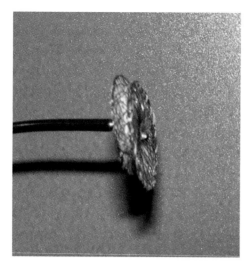

Figure 16.12 The Amplatzer perimembranous ventricular septal defect device. The two discs are offset from each other to minimise the chance of the left ventricular disc impinging on the aortic valve. The central stent is much narrower than in the muscular ventricular septal defect device as the membranous septum is much thinner than the muscular septum.

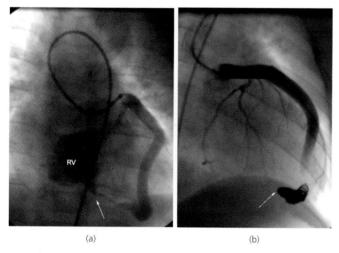

(a)   (b)

Figure 16.13 Coil occlusion of a coronary fistula. A selective left coronary arteriogram shows a fistula arising from the left anterior descending coronary artery (arrow, (a)) draining to the right ventricle (RV). Multiple interlocking detachable coils are placed to completely occlude the fistula (arrow, (b)).

Other procedures

Coils and Amplatzer patent ductus arteriosus devices have been used to occlude prosthetic paravalvar leaks, ruptured aneurysms of the sinus of Valsalva and other fistulae (Figure 16.13) with good

success. Amplatzer atrial septal defect devices have been used for pseudoaneurysms of the ascending and descending aorta.

Percutaneous intervention and surgery

The growth of interventional cardiology has meant that the simpler defects are now dealt with in catheterisation laboratories, and cardiac surgeons are increasingly operating on more complex lesions such as hypoplastic left heart syndrome. More importantly, interventional cardiology can complement the management of patients with these complex lesions, resulting in a better outcome for children with congenital heart disease.

In some conditions, the surgeon and the interventionalist can work together to achieve the desired outcome. These hybrid procedures include perventricular ventricular septal defect closure, intra-operative pulmonary artery stenting and branch pulmonary artery banding with stenting of the arterial duct used to palliate neonates with hypoplastic left heart syndrome. Collaboration in this setting provides the interventionalist with direct access to the heart and avoids the need for cardiopulmonary bypass. This collaboration includes preparation of the heart by the surgeon for transcatheter completion of total cavopulmonary circulation with a covered stent from the inferior vena cava to the pulmonary artery. Such cooperation is likely to provide a cornerstone of patient management in the future of paediatric cardiology.

Further reading

Carminati M, Butera G, Chessa M *et al*. Transcatheter closure of congenital ventricular septal defects: results of the European registry. *Eur Heart J* 2007;**28**:2361–8.

Kan JS, White RI Jr, Mitchell SE, Gardner TJ. Percutaneous balloon valvuloplasty: a new method for treating congenital pulmonary valve stenosis. *N Engl J Med* 1982;**307**:540–2.

Masura J, Walsh KP, Thanopoulous B *et al*. Catheter closure of moderate- to large-sized patent ductus arteriosus using the new Amplatzer duct occluder: immediate and short-term results. *J Am Coll Cardiol* 1998;**31**:878–82.

Morrison WL, Walsh KP. Transcatheter closure of ventricular septal defect post myocardial infarction. In: Grech ED, Ramsdale DR, eds. *Practical Interventional Cardiology*. 2nd ed. London: Martin Dunitz, 2002:362–64.

Mullins CE. *Cardiac Catheterization in Congenital Heart Disease*. Malden, Massachusetts: Blackwell Publishing, 2006.

Waight DJ, Cao Q-L, Hijazi ZM. Interventional cardiac catheterisation in adults with congenital heart disease. In: Grech ED, Ramsdale DR, eds. *Practical Interventional Cardiology*. 2nd ed. London: Martin Dunitz, 2002:390–406.

Walsh KP, Maadi IM. The Amplatzer septal occluder. *Cardiol Young* 2000;**10**:493–501.

Index

Note: Page numbers in *italics* refer to figures, those in **bold** refer to tables

CURRENT TITLES

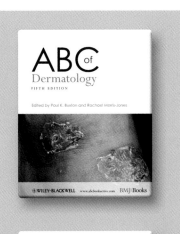

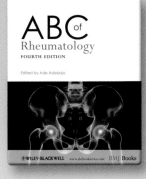

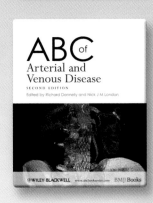

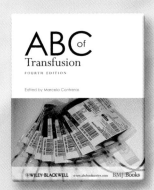

ABC of Dermatology
5TH EDITION

Edited by Paul K. Buxton & Rachael Morris-Jones
Consultant Dermatologist, Hampshire; King's College Hospital, London

- A new 20th anniversary edition of this bestselling *ABC* covering the diagnosis and treatment of skin conditions for the non-dermatologist
- Covers the core knowledge on therapy, management and diagnosis of common conditions and highlights the evidence base
- Provides clear learning outcomes and basic science boxes
- Includes a new chapter on the general principles of skin condition management for specialist nurses

March 2009 | 9781405170659 | 224 pages
£28.99/US$52.95/€35.90/AU$57.95

ABC of Rheumatology
4TH EDITION

Edited by Ade Adebajo
University of Sheffield

- A practical guide to the diagnosis and treatment of rheumatology for the non-specialist
- Fully revised and updated to include information on new treatments and therapies while covering the core knowledge on therapy, management and diagnosis
- A highly illustrated, informative and practical source of knowledge offering links to further information and resources
- This established *ABC* is an accessible reference for all primary care health professionals

October 2009 | 9781405170680 | 192 pages
£27.99/US$44.95/€34.90/AU$57.95

ABC of Arterial and Venous Disease
2ND EDITION

Edited by Richard Donnelly & Nick J.M. London
University of Nottingham; University of Leicester

- A practical guide to the diagnosis and treatment of arterial and venous disease for the non-specialist, focusing on the modern day management of patients
- Explains the different interventions for arterial and venous disease
- Covers the core knowledge on therapy, management and diagnosis and highlights the evidence base on varicose veins, diabetes, blood clots, stroke and TIA and use of stents
- This revised new edition now includes information on new treatments and therapies, antithrombotic therapy, and non-invasive techniques

April 2009 | 9781405178891 | 120 pages
£26.99/US$49.95/€33.90/AU$54.95

ABC of Transfusion
4TH EDITION

Edited by Marcela Contreras
Royal Free and University College Hospitals Medical School, London

- A comprehensive and highly regarded guide to all the practical aspects of blood transfusion
- This new edition is an established reference from a leading centre in transfusion
- Includes five new chapters on variant CJD, stem cell transplantation, immunotherapy, blood matching and appropriate use of transfusion
- Reflects the latest developments in blood transfusion management

March 2009 | 9781405156462 | 128 pages
£26.99/US$49.95/€33.90/AU$54.95

For more information on any of the titles, please visit the *ABC* website at **www.abcbookseries.com**

CURRENT TITLES

ABC of Mental Health
2ND EDITION

Edited by Teifion Davies & Tom Craig
Both King's College, London Institute of Psychiatry

- Provides clear practical advice on how to recognise, diagnose and manage mental disorders successfully and safely

- Includes sections on selecting drugs and psychological treatments, and improving compliance

- Contains information on the major categories of mental health disorders, the mental health needs of vulnerable groups (such as the elderly, children, homeless and ethnic minorities) and psychological treatments

- Covers the mental health needs of special groups: equips GPs and hospital doctors with all the information they need for the day to day management of patients with mental health problems

May 2009 | 9780727916396 | 128 pages
£27.99/US$47.95/€34.90/AU$57.95

ABC of Lung Cancer

Edited by Ian Hunt, Martin M. Muers & Tom Treasure
Guy's Hospital, London; Leeds General Infirmary; Guy's & St. Thomas' Hospital, London

- A practical guide for those involved in the care of the lung cancer patient

- An up-to-date evidence-based review of one of the most common cancers in the western world

- Written by the specialists involved in the launch of the NICE UK Lung Cancer Guidelines

- Looks at the epidemiology and diagnosis of lung cancer, focusing particularly on primary care issues

April 2009 | 9781405146524 | 64 pages
£21.99/US$37.95/€27.90/AU$44.95

ABC of Spinal Disorders

Edited by Andrew Clarke, Alwyn Jones, Michael O'Malley & Robert McLaren
Royal Devon and Exeter Hospital; University of Wales Hospital, Cardiff; Warrington Hospital; GP

- This brand new title addresses the causes and management of the different spinal conditions presenting in general practice

- Provides much needed practical guidance on the diagnosis, treatment and advice as back pain is one of the commonest causes for absence from work and is a chronic problem confronting general practitioners

- Includes guidance for the GP when they have to refer patients for more specialist treatment

December 2009 | 9781405170697 | 72 pages
£19.99/US$35.95/€24.90/AU$39.95

ABC of Medical Law

Lorraine Corfield, Ingrid Granne & William Latimer-Sayer
Guy's and St Thomas' NHS Trust, London; University of Oxford; Lawyer, Clinical Negligence and Personal Injury Specialist

- Fills the gap for a basic introduction to legal issues in health care that is easy to understand and act upon

- Provides up to date coverage of contentious issues such as withholding and withdrawing treatment and confidentiality

- Accessible to those without any legal knowledge, providing guidance without becoming embroiled in complicated legal discussion

June 2009 | 9781405176286 | 64 pages
£19.99/US$35.95/€24.90/AU$39.95

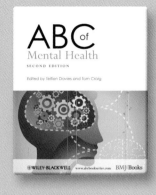
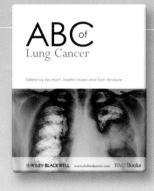
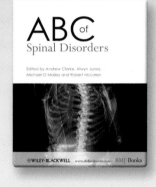
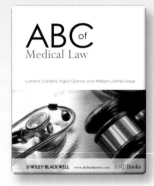

For more information on any of our medical books, please visit **www.wiley.com/go/medicine**

CURRENT TITLES

ABC of the First Year
6TH EDITION

Bernard Valman & Roslyn Thomas
Both Northwick Park Hospital, Harrow, Middlesex

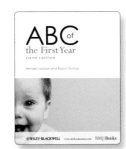

- Includes new sections on recognition and prevention of obesity in weaning, and good weaning practices
- Helps practitioners answer parents and carers questions about what's normal and what's a concern
- Includes a Development Chart (up to 2 years of age) showing the normal range and different cut-offs, in different abilities or activities
- Features recommendations that conform to the latest NICE guidelines
- Includes useful links and addresses such as patient resources and organisations

January 2009 | 9781405180375 | 136 pages | £26.99/US$49.95/€33.90/AU$54.95

ABC of One to Seven
5TH EDITION

Edited by Bernard Valman
Northwick Park Hospital, Harrow, Middlesex

- Provides a guide to the diseases, developmental disorders, and emotional problems of early childhood
- Each chapter contains concise advice on the child health problems most frequently encountered by primary health care workers
- Includes new chapters on prevention and management of obesity, immunisation, and a section on ADHD and autism with guidance on what to refer and when, and how to manage afterwards
- Includes a Development Chart, covering the full age range, showing the normal range and different cut-offs, in different abilities and activities
- Includes an appendix of patient resources including links to organisations, the department of health and the Royal Colleges, and a chapter explaining NHS direct and changes to legislation for social services following the Children Act

October 2009 | 9781405181051 | 168 pages | £27.99/US$47.95/€34.90/AU$57.95

ABC of Geriatric Medicine

Edited by Nicola Cooper, Kirsty Forrest & Graham Mulley
Leeds General Infirmary; Leeds Teaching Hospital NHS Trust; St James's University Hospital, Leeds

- A practical guide for all who care for older people
- Provides an overview of key topics in geriatric medicine with references, further reading and resources
- Based on the UK specialty training curriculum in geriatric medicine

January 2009 | 9781405169424 | 88 pages | £21.99/US$39.95/€27.90/AU$44.95

ABC of Emergency Differential Diagnosis

Edited by Francis Morris & Alan Fletcher
Both Northern General Hospital, Sheffield

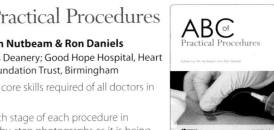

- A practical, step-by-step guide to the diagnosis and treatment of acute conditions for non-specialists
- Covers the essentials on symptoms, assessment, diagnosis, treatment and management of the most important conditions
- Includes 'walk-through' diagnosis, clear learning outcomes, and easy to find treatment options
- Takes a problem-based approach for the rapid assimilation of information
- Features case studies that allow the reader to be sure that they have synthesised the information given and can apply it to clinical cases

July 2009 | 9781405170635 | 96 pages | £26.99/US$49.95/€32.90/AU$54.95

ABC of Practical Procedures

Edited by Tim Nutbeam & Ron Daniels
West Midlands Deanery; Good Hope Hospital, Heart of England Foundation Trust, Birmingham

- Teaches the core skills required of all doctors in training
- Features each stage of each procedure in colour step-by-step photographs as it is being performed
- Features a useful tips/handy hints box to aid key skills learning

November 2009 | 9781405185950 | 144 pages | £25.99/US$44.95/€31.90/AU$52.95

ABC of Sepsis

Edited by Ron Daniels & Tim Nutbeam
Good Hope Hospital, Heart of England Foundation Trust, Birmingham, Surviving Sepsis Campaign UK and Survive Sepsis; West Midlands Deanery and Survive Sepsis

- A much needed introduction to this important subject - a core aspect of acute medicine in the UK
- Offers a basic introduction to sepsis for trainees and the MDT
- A timely subject due to current concerns regarding hospital infection and patient safety
- The authors are involved with the Surviving Sepsis campaign, developed to improve the management, diagnosis and treatment of sepsis

December 2009 | 9781405181945 | 104 pages | £25.99/US$46.95/€32.90/AU$52.95

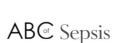

For more information on any of the titles, please visit the *ABC* website at **www.abcbookseries.com**

ALSO AVAILABLE

ABC of Adolescence
Russell Viner
2005 | 9780727915740 | 56 pages | £22.99/US$37.95/€28.90/AU$47.95

ABC of Allergies
Stephen R. Durham
1998 | 9780727912367 | 65 pages | £25.99/US$47.95/€32.90/AU$52.95

ABC of Antenatal Care, 4th Edition
Geoffrey Chamberlain & Margery Morgan
2002 | 9780727916921 | 92 pages | £23.99/US$44.95/€29.90/AU$47.95

ABC of Antithrombotic Therapy
Gregory Y.H. Lip & Andrew D. Blann
2003 | 9780727917713 | 67 pages | £21.99/US$37.95/€27.90/AU$44.95

ABC of Brain Stem Death, 2nd Edition
Christopher Pallis & D.H. Harley
1996 | 9780727902450 | 55 pages | £26.99/US$49.95/€32.90/AU$54.95

ABC of Breast Diseases, 3rd Edition
J. Michael Dixon
2005 | 9780727918284 | 120 pages | £28.99/US$53.95/€35.90/AU$57.95

ABC of Burns
Shehan Hettiaratchy, Remo Papini & Peter Dziewulski
2004 | 9780727917874 | 56 pages | £21.99/US$37.95/€27.90/AU$44.95

ABC of Child Protection, 4th Edition
Sir Roy Meadow, Jacqueline Mok & Donna Rosenberg
2007 | 9780727918178 | 120 pages | £28.99/US$53.95/€34.90/AU$57.95

ABC of Clinical Electrocardiography, 2nd Edition
Francis Morris, William Brady & John Camm
2008 | 9781405170642 | 112 pages | £27.99/US$52.95/€34.90/AU$57.95

ABC of Clinical Genetics, 3rd Edition
Helen M. Kingston
2002 | 9780727916273 | 120 pages | £26.99/US$50.95/€33.90/AU$54.95

ABC of Clinical Haematology, 3rd Edition
Drew Provan
2007 | 9781405153539 | 112 pages | £28.99/US$53.95/€35.90/AU$57.95

ABC of Colorectal Diseases, 2nd Edition
David Jones
1998 | 9780727911056 | 110 pages | £28.99/US$53.95/€34.90/AU$57.95

ABC of Complementary Medicine, 2nd Edition
Catherine Zollman, Andrew Vickers & Janet Richardson
2008 | 9781405136570 | 58 pages | £22.99/US$42.95/€28.90/AU$47.95

ABC of Conflict and Disaster
Anthony Redmond, Peter F. Mahoney, James Ryan, Cara Macnab & Lord David Owen
2005 | 9780727917263 | 80 pages | £21.99/US$37.95/€27.90/AU$44.95

ABC of COPD
Graeme P. Currie
2006 | 9781405147118 | 48 pages | £21.99/US$37.95/€27.90/AU$44.95

ABC of Ear, Nose and Throat, 5th Edition
Harold S. Ludman & Patrick Bradley
2007 | 9781405136563 | 120 pages | £28.99/US$53.95/€35.90/AU$57.95

ABC of Eating Disorders
Jane Morris
2008 | 9780727918437 | 80 pages | £21.99/US$37.95/€27.90/AU$44.95

ABC of Emergency Radiology, 2nd Edition
Otto Chan
2007 | 9780727915283 | 144 pages | £29.99/US$53.95/€36.90/AU$59.95

ABC of Eyes, 4th Edition
Peng T. Khaw, Peter Shah & Andrew R. Elkington
2004 | 9780727916594 | 104 pages | £27.99/US$49.95/€34.90/AU$57.95

ABC of Headache
Anne MacGregor & Alison Frith
2008 | 9781405170666 | 88 pages | £21.99/US$37.95/€27.90/AU$44.95

ABC of Health Informatics
Frank Sullivan & Jeremy Wyatt
2006 | 9780727918505 | 56 pages | £21.99/US$37.95/€27.90/AU$44.95

ABC of Heart Failure, 2nd Edition
Russell C. Davis, Michael K. Davies & Gregory Y.H. Lip
2006 | 9780727916440 | 72 pages | £21.99/US$37.95/€27.90/AU$44.95

ABC of Hypertension, 5th Edition
Gareth Beevers, Gregory Y.H. Lip & Eoin O'Brien
2007 | 9781405130615 | 88 pages | £26.99/US$47.95/€32.90/AU$54.95

ABC of Interventional Cardiology
Ever D. Grech
2003 | 9780727915467 | 51 pages | £21.99/US$37.95/€27.90/AU$44.95

ABC of Kidney Disease
David Goldsmith, Satishkumar Abeythunge Jayawardene & Penny Ackland
2007 | 9781405136754 | 96 pages | £27.99/US$52.95/€34.90/AU$57.95

ABC of Labour Care
Geoffrey Chamberlain, Philip Steer & Luke Zander
1999 | 9780727914156 | 60 pages | £19.99/US$35.95/€24.90/AU$39.95

ABC of Liver, Pancreas and Gall Bladder
Ian Beckingham
2001 | 9780727915313 | 64 pages | £19.99/US$35.95/€24.90/AU$39.95

ABC of Major Trauma, 3rd Edition
Peter Driscoll, David Skinner & Richard Earlam
1999 | 9780727913784 | 192 pages | £25.99/US$49.95/€31.90/AU$52.95

ABC of Monitoring Drug Therapy
Jeffrey Aronson, M. Hardman & D.J.M. Reynolds
1993 | 9780727907912 | 46 pages | £21.99/US$37.95/€27.90/AU$44.95

ABC of Nutrition, 4th Edition
A. Stewart Truswell
2003 | 9780727916648 | 152 pages | £26.99/US$49.95/€32.90/AU$54.95

ABC of Obesity
Naveed Sattar & Mike Lean
2007 | 9781405136747 | 64 pages | £21.99/US$35.95/€27.90/AU$44.95

ABC of Occupational and Environmental Medicine, 2nd Edition
David Snashall & Dipti Patel
2003 | 9780727916112 | 124 pages | £28.99/US$53.95/€35.90/AU$57.95

ABC of Oral Health
Crispian Scully
2000 | 9780727915511 | 41 pages | £19.99/US$35.95/€24.90/AU$39.95

ABC of Palliative Care, 2nd Edition
Marie Fallon & Geoffrey Hanks
2006 | 9781405130790 | 96 pages | £24.99/US$47.95/€30.90/AU$49.95

ABC of Patient Safety
John Sandars & Gary Cook
2007 | 9781405156929 | 64 pages | £23.99/US$42.95/€29.90/AU$47.95

ABC of Preterm Birth
William McGuire & Peter Fowlie
2005 | 9780727917638 | 56 pages | £21.99/US$37.95/€27.90/AU$44.95

ABC of Psychological Medicine
Richard Mayou, Michael Sharpe & Alan Carson
2003 | 9780727915566 | 72 pages | £22.99/US$37.95/€27.90/AU$47.95

ABC of Resuscitation, 5th Edition
Michael Colquhoun, Anthony Handley & T.R. Evans
2003 | 9780727916693 | 111 pages | £28.99/US$53.95/€34.90/AU$57.95

ABC of Sexual Health, 2nd Edition
John Tomlinson
2004 | 9780727917591 | 96 pages | £25.99/US$47.95/€32.90/AU$52.95

ABC of Sexually Transmitted Infections, 5th Edition
Michael W. Adler, Frances Cowan, Patrick French, Helen Mitchell & John Richens
2004 | 9780727917614 | 104 pages | £25.99/US$49.95/€31.90/AU$52.95

ABC of Skin Cancer
Sajjad Rajpar & Jerry Marsden
2008 | 9781405162197 | 80 pages | £21.99/US$41.95/€27.90/AU$44.95

ABC of Smoking Cessation
John Britton
2004 | 9780727918185 | 56 pages | £18.99/US$35.95/€22.90/AU$37.95

ABC of Sports and Exercise Medicine, 3rd Edition
Gregory Whyte, Mark Harries & Clyde Williams
2005 | 9780727918130 | 136 pages | £28.99/US$56.95/€34.90/AU$57.95

ABC of Subfertility
Peter Braude & Alison Taylor
2004 | 9780727915344 | 64 pages | £19.99/US$35.95/€24.90/AU$39.95

ABC of Tubes, Drains, Lines and Frames
Adam Brooks, Peter F. Mahoney & Brian Rowlands
2008 | 9781405160148 | 88 pages | £21.99/US$37.95/€27.90/AU$44.95

ABC of the Upper Gastrointestinal Tract
Robert Logan, Adam Harris, J.J. Misiewicz & J.H. Baron
2002 | 9780727912664 | 54 pages | £21.99/US$37.95/€27.90/AU$44.95

ABC of Urology, 2nd Edition
Chris Dawson & Hugh N. Whitfield
2006 | 9781405139595 | 64 pages | £22.99/US$42.95/€27.90/AU$47.95

ABC of Wound Healing
Joseph E. Grey & Keith G. Harding
2006 | 9780727916952 | 56 pages | £21.99/US$37.95/€27.90/AU$44.95